Lessons From
A Horse Named Jim

A Clinical Trials Manual
From The Duke Clinical Research Institute

by Margaret B. Liu and Kate Davis

Published by the Duke Clinical Research Institute
3708 Mayfair Street, Durham NC 27707

ISBN: 0-9712529-0-4

Printed in the United States of America

Table of Contents

Preface

We are members of a small unique group within the Duke Clinical Research Institute (DCRI) who develop instructional materials to help site personnel conduct clinical trials efficiently. Our work led us to become involved with multiple trial teams within the DCRI and with a variety of sponsors. As a result, we noticed that individuals used the lingo and acronyms of clinical research without fully understanding the meaning and how to apply the general information to a specific trial. Fact and fiction were inter-mixed, and there was no readily available resource to demystify the world of clinical research.

Fortunately, circumstances allowed us to pursue our dream of creating a user-friendly manual that could be a resource for principal investigators and study coordinators. We were able to spend the hours needed to write and rewrite the book that ultimately met our needs.

The first half of the manual is organized into chapters that provide the historical framework, the rules and regulations, definitions, and necessary oversight of clinical trials. The remaining chapters focus on how clinical trials are conducted at the investigative sites, with an emphasis on the practical application of the information presented in the first half. These later chapters not only give tips on organizing and conducting clinical trials at the site, but also provide examples of forms and documents that might be used in a clinical trial.

This book would not have been possible without the insight of those who challenged processes or operating procedures and asked for clarification. We gathered information from many talented and experienced DCRI employees as well as from external colleagues with whom we established relationships over the years. Some of our colleagues reviewed chapters while others contributed through brainstorming meetings and hallway discussions. We would like to thank Alice Brunk, Arleen Eppinger, Lisa Berdan, John Alexander, Anne Holland, Pam Tenaerts, Jean Bolte, Sharon Karnash, and Ken Ross for their insightful comments on our earliest version. Several others contributed to subsequent versions, including Patty McAdams, Julie Szabo, Bert Hinman-Smith, Mike Cuffe, Kristina Sigmon, Amanda Stebbins, Bunny Donohue, Cindy Gordon, Gail Fowler, and Francie Seymour. Benetta Walker and Lisa Zimmerman helped us better understand the practical application of the regulations, and John Daniel, Penny Hodgson, Jenny Walker, and Pat French provided us with editorial support. Finally, Joy Mickle and Kerry Bassett took our printed words and converted them to a highly readable and interesting format, while Beth Carlton took care of getting the manual into print. We are grateful to all of them and to still others who provided us with encouragement when we could not see the light at the end of the tunnel. This book could not have been completed without their help and support.

—*Margaret B. Liu and Kate Davis*

Introduction

While much has been written about the theory behind the design of clinical trials and the statistical and clinical interpretation of the results, little has been written about the process of conducting trials. For too long there has been a dissociation between the theory and the practice of clinical research. This manual is intended to be one step towards bridging that gap. By combining sound fundamental practices of clinical research with good research ideas in the right clinical environment, we can continue to make advances that will improve the lives of the patients we serve.

From its inception the Duke Clinical Research Institute (DCRI) has had a mission: to develop and share knowledge that improves the care of patients around the world through innovative clinical research. Our "bottom line" is to save patients' lives and improve their quality of life by offering clinicians new information about the best ways to care for their patients. We strive to accomplish this by designing and conducting clinical trials and outcome studies that provide the answers to important medical questions about patient care.

With the publication of this manual, a long-time goal of many people who work at the DCRI has been realized. Early in our experience coordinating clinical trials, we recognized the need to pull together information related to the pragmatic conduct of clinical trials and organize it logically into one reference manual. Our hope has been to have this information at our fingertips in order to quickly and accurately share it with our staff, the staff of our collaborating coordinating centers, and site personnel participating in the trials we coordinate. By placing our views of clinical research methodology in printed form, we hope not only to influence the use of medical therapies, but also to improve the system that delivers the evidence needed for this era of evidence-based medicine. While Ms. Liu and Ms. Davis deserve great credit for putting the manual together, it truly represents the joint effort of hundreds of DCRI employees and collaborators in the academic, industry and government worlds.

—*Robert M. Califf, MD*

ABBREVIATIONS

ARO   Academic Research Organization

ADE   Adverse Drug Experience

ADR   Adverse Drug Reaction

AE   Adverse Event

CFR   Code of Federal Regulations

CRF   Case Report Form

CRO   Contract Research Organization

DSMB   Data and Safety Monitoring Board

FDA   Food and Drug Administration

GCP   Good Clinical Practice

GLP   Good Laboratory Practice

GMP   Good Manufacturing Practice

ICH   International Conference on Harmonization

IDE   Investigational Device Exemption

IND   Investigational New Drug Application

IRB   Institutional Review Board

NDA   New Drug Application

PI   Principal Investigator

SAE   Serious Adverse Event

SMO   Site Management Organization

SOP   Standard Operating Procedure

GLOSSARY

Academic Research Organization (ARO)   An academic organization that sponsors a trial or is contracted by the sponsor to perform one or more of a sponsor's trial-related activities, including but not limited to: protocol development and design, recruitment of investigators, study management and coordination, monitoring, data management, and statistical analysis. An ARO uses academic leaders and/or clinicians to provide leadership and may be affiliated with an academic institution.

Adverse Drug Reaction (ADR)   A response to an *investigational drug* that occurs at any dose and is noxious and unintended. A response to a *marketed drug* that is noxious, unintended, and that occurs at doses normally used for prophylaxis, diagnosis, therapy, or for modification of physiological function. Adverse drug reactions can be *expected* or *unexpected*.

Adverse Event (AE)   Any unfavorable change that may affect a subject during or after a clinical trial; the change is not necessarily caused by the investigational product. Includes physical signs and symptoms, abnormal laboratory findings, changes in vital signs, a new condition or illness, or the worsening of a condition or illness that was present before product use. Also called *adverse experience*. When a causal relationship has been established between a product and the AE, the AE is referred to as an adverse drug reaction (causal relationship with a drug) or an adverse device effect (causal relationship with a medical device).

Amendment   See *Protocol Amendment*.

Assent   An agreement to participate in clinical research. Assent may be required from children who are of adequate age and emotional maturity to understand the concept of the study but are incapable of grasping all the details of the study.

Assurance   A legally binding written document that requires a public or private institution to comply with applicable federal minimum standards for the protection of human subjects in research.

Audit   An independent and systematic review of study data, associated records, protocol procedures, study conduct, and interim or final study reports to determine whether the information is accurate and whether the study has been carried out in compliance with the protocol, standard operating procedures, good clinical practice, and applicable regulations. Sponsors may conduct internal audits, audits of AROs/CROs designated to perform sponsor responsibilities, and audits of investigative sites participating in a clinical trial. Audits may also be performed to review manufacturing practices, laboratory processes, and storage facilities.

Audit Trail   Documentation of events that allows auditors to identify the original source of the data and track the path of changes made to the original documentation.

Belmont Report   Report issued by the National Commission for the Protection of Human Subjects of Biomedical and Behavioral Research. The Belmont Report identifies basic ethical principles for the conduct of clinical research.

Benefit   A valued, favorable, or desired outcome.

Blinding   A procedure in which one or more parties in a clinical trial are kept unaware of the treatment assignments. In a *single-blind* study, the subjects are unaware of the treatment assignments, while in a *double-blind* study, the subjects, investigators, and study personnel are unaware of the treatment assignments. In case of emergencies that require knowledge of the treatment assignment, mechanisms exist to *unblind* the code, commonly called *breaking the blind*. An open or open label study has no blinding of the subject or the study staff.

Case Report Form (CRF)   A printed, optical, or electronic document used to record protocol-required information for each subject in the study.

Causality Assessment   A determination of whether an adverse event may have been caused by or related to an investigational product. Examples of categories for causality include: (1) *not a reasonable possibility*—it is unlikely the adverse event was caused by the investigational product, and (2) *a reasonable possibility*—the adverse event may have been caused by the investigational product. Further categorization sometimes includes (1) unrelated, (2) remotely related, (3) possibly related, (4) probably related, and (5) definitely related.

Children (in clinical research)   Individuals who are under the legal age to give consent for participation in a clinical research study. The assent of children who are considered of adequate age and emotional maturity may be required for study participation. Specific legal age is determined under the applicable laws in the jurisdiction where the research is being conducted.

Clinical Trial   Systematic study conducted in human subjects.

Code of Federal Regulations (CFR)   An annually revised documentation of the general and permanent rules published in the Federal Register. The code is divided into 50 titles that represent broad areas subject to federal regulations. Title 21 of the CFR includes most of the regulations affecting the discovery, development, approval, and marketing of drugs and devices.

Coding   Assigning data such as adverse events and medications to categories. This allows data to be grouped and retrieved for analysis. Codes may be a group of letters, numbers, or symbols with associated rules for usage.

Compliance   Adherence to protocol requirements, standards of good clinical practice, and applicable regulations.

Confidentiality   Prevention of unauthorized disclosure of a sponsor's proprietary information or of a subject's identity and personal medical information.

Contract Research Organization (CRO)   An organization contracted by the sponsor to perform one or more of a sponsor's trial-related activities, including but not limited to: protocol development and design, recruitment of investigators, study management and coordination, monitoring, data management, and statistical analysis. Compare to Academic Research Organization (ARO).

Consent Form   See *Informed Consent*.

Control Group   The group of patients who receive the standard treatment (no treatment or placebo) and who are compared to the group of patients receiving the investigational treatment.

Curriculum Vitae (CV)   A summary of an investigator's education, training, and experience; similar to a resume.

Data and Safety Monitoring Board (DSMB)   An independent committee of clinicians, statisticians, ethicists, and other specialists who assess the progress of a trial, its safety, and its efficacy at specified intervals. The committee can make recommendations that a study be continued, modified, or stopped based on the data reviewed.

Data Forms   Forms used to record patient data from original source documents. Including but not limited to: case report forms, enrollment forms, serious adverse event forms, and follow-up forms. Also referred to as *patient data forms*.

Declaration of Helsinki   A statement of ethical principles developed by the 18th World Medical Assembly, Helsinki, Finland, June 1964, to provide guidance to physicians who practice biomedical research involving human subjects. The declaration sets forth the requirements for the ethical treatment of patients and research volunteers. It mandates obtaining informed consent and stresses the overriding importance of the subjects' needs as individuals over the needs of science and society. The basic thrust of the Declaration of Helsinki is incorporated in the Code of Federal Regulations (21 § CFR 312).

Double-Blind Study   See *Blinding*.

Drug Accountability   Records of the receipt and disposition of investigational drug supplies.

Eligibility Criteria   Rules for selecting subjects to participate in a clinical trial. Participants must meet all of the inclusion criteria for trial entry and not have any of the exclusion criteria.

Endpoint   An indicator measured to assess the effect of a treatment or therapy—an assessment of safety, efficacy, or another study objective. Also called *outcome, variable, parameter, marker, and measure*.

Equipoise   The state resulting from the presumed equality of the study treatments. In this situation, an investigator may be uncertain about which study treatment would be more beneficial for a patient.

Exclusion Criteria   Rules of eligibility that exclude an individual from participation in a study.

Expedited Adverse Event Reporting   Reporting of adverse events designated by the protocol/sponsor to the FDA within specified time frames.

Federal Register   A weekly publication that identifies proposed and approved regulations.

Food and Drug Administration (FDA)   A division of the Department of Health and Human Services responsible for assuring the safety and efficacy of pharmaceuticals, biological products, and medical devices, and the safety of foods and cosmetics. Primary FDA offices are located in Rockville, Maryland; the internet address is www.fda.gov.

Form FDA 1571   The Investigational New Drug (IND) application form that is completed and submitted by the sponsor as part of the IND application.

Form FDA 1572   This *Statement of Investigator* form must be completed by all investigators participating in a clinical trial when an Investigational New Drug (IND) application is being submitted or an existing IND is being updated. By signing this form, the investigator agrees to comply with all regulations pertaining to clinical research. The completed and signed form is submitted to the sponsor, who in turn submits it to the FDA.

Good Clinical Practice (GCP)   The standards for the design, conduct, performance, monitoring, auditing, recording, analyses, and reporting of clinical trials. These standards provide assurance that the data and reported results are credible and accurate, and that the rights, integrity, and confidentiality of trial subjects are protected.

Good Laboratory Practice (GLP)   Regulations found in Title 21, Part 58, that apply to clinical laboratories performing analyses for clinical trials. Key provisions of Good Laboratory Practice regulations are requirements for creating a quality assurance unit; developing standard operating procedures; analyzing of the investigational product for concentration, uniformity, and stability; and the maintaining, calibrating, and standardizing instruments.

Good Manufacturing Practice (GMP)   Regulations found in Title 21, Parts 210, 211, and 820. GMP regulations describe the methods, equipment, facilities, and controls required for producing products, devices, and food. The regulations apply to clinical research when pharmaceutical products and medical devices are manufactured and tested, and they apply to any drug product intended for administration to humans or animals, including products still in developmental stages.

Guidelines   Written principles and practices pertaining to applying the regulations. Although guidelines are an accepted standard of practice, they are not enforceable by law. *FDA guidelines* are applicable in the United States while *International Conference on Harmonization (ICH) guidelines* reflect an international movement to standardize practices across national borders.

Inclusion Criteria   Rules of eligibility that an individual must meet in order to participate in a clinical study. See Eligibility Criteria.

Informed Consent   A process by which a subject voluntarily confirms his or her willingness to participate in a clinical trial after having been informed of all aspects relevant to the subject's decision to participate. The Declaration of Helsinki states that in any human research, each potential subject must be adequately informed of the aims, methods, anticipated benefits, potential hazards, and discomforts that study participation might entail. Informed consent is typically documented via a written, signed, and dated *consent form*.

Inspection   An official review by regulatory authorities of documents, facilities, records, and other study-related resources. Inspections may be carried out at investigative sites, at the facilities of the sponsor, at organizations performing sponsor-delegated activities, or at other establishments deemed appropriate by the authorities performing the inspection.

Institutional Review Board (IRB)   A board, committee, or other group that reviews and approves clinical studies at an investigative site. The primary responsibility of the committee is to ensure the protection of the rights and welfare of study participants. Also called *Independent Review Committee, Ethics Committee, Human Protection Committee*.

International Conference on Harmonization (ICH) A committee established to develop a unified standard for the European Union, Japan, and the United States, and to facilitate the mutual acceptance of clinical data by regulatory authorities in these jurisdictions.

Investigational Device Exemption (IDE) Exemption from certain regulatory requirements that apply to commercially distributed medical devices in order to allow manufacturers to distribute devices that are intended solely for investigational use on human subjects. An approved IDE application permits a device that would otherwise be subject to marketing clearance to be lawfully shipped for use in a clinical study.

Investigational New Drug (IND) Application An application that sponsors must submit to the FDA before beginning studies of an investigational drug in humans. An IND is an application for exemption from the laws that prevent the distribution and use of pharmaceutical agents that have not been approved for use by the FDA. The IND should describe the plan for treatment, previous human experience with the investigational drug, the structural formula, animal test results, and manufacturing information. Also called the *Notice of Claimed Investigational Exemption for a New Drug*.

Investigational New Drug (IND) Safety Report A report issued by the sponsor of an investigational product when a safety issue arises. The report is submitted to the FDA and to investigators participating in the clinical trial.

Investigative Site The location where a study is being conducted. Site locations include physicians' offices, hospitals, and outpatient clinics. Also known as *study site*.

Investigator An individual who conducts a clinical study and directs the use, administration, and distribution of the investigational agent to a subject. When a team of individuals at a specific location conducts an investigation, the investigator is the responsible leader of the group. The investigator holds regulatory responsibility for the conduct of the trial at the investigative site. A *co-investigator* is an individual who shares equal responsibility in conducting the trial at a site.

Investigator-Directed Inspection An FDA inspection that focuses on the work of an investigator rather than on a specific study. This may be an extension of a study-directed inspection and may result from problems encountered during, or questions arising from, a study-directed inspection. Formerly referred to as *for-cause inspection*; also see *Inspection*.

Investigator's Brochure A brochure compiled by the sponsor providing all known information about the test article or investigational agent. It includes the formulation of the investigational agent, pharmacology, toxicology, pharmacokinetics, safety and effectiveness data, possible side effects, and risks. Both pre-clinical and clinical data are included. Also called *investigator's drug brochure* and *investigational drug brochure*.

Letter of Agreement   A letter outlining the terms of the contract between the sponsor and an investigator. Contents of a letter of agreement usually include the terms of the study, including the start and anticipated end of the study, payment methods, data confidentiality, publishing requirements, and product liability issues.

Letter of Indemnification   A legal document indicating protection or exemption from liability. The letter of indemnification usually protects the investigator and investigative site from claims by the study participant that harm was caused as a result of participation in the clinical trial. It does not, however, protect the investigator from claims resulting from negligence on the part of the investigator.

Monitor   An individual selected by a sponsor to oversee the progress of a clinical investigation. Activities often include site visits to ensure that the investigator is fulfilling the responsibilities set forth in the Code of Federal Regulations, that the data submitted are accurate and complete, and that regulatory requirements pertaining to protocol compliance, adverse event reporting, IRB review and approval, and informed consent are met. Also known as *Clinical Research Associate (CRA)* and *Clinical Trial Monitor (CTM)*.

Monitoring   Overseeing the progress of a clinical trial to ensure that it is conducted, recorded, and reported according to the protocol, standard operating procedures, good clinical practice guidelines, and applicable regulations.

New Drug Application (NDA)   An application submitted to the FDA requesting approval to market a new drug for human use. The contents of the NDA are provided to demonstrate the safety and efficacy of the investigational drug. The application contains information about the class of the drug, the scientific rationale for the drug, its intended use, and the potential clinical benefits. A summary of the clinical data collected is included with the results of the statistical analyses of the clinical trials.

Nuremberg Code   A code of ethics developed from the Nuremberg Military Tribunal's decision in the case of the *US versus Karl Brandt, et al*. The Code includes ten conditions delineating permissible medical experimentation on human subjects. According to this code, human experimentation is justified only if its results benefit society and if it is carried out in accord with the basic principles that "satisfy moral, ethical, and legal concepts."

Open-Label Study   A study in which the treatment assignment is not blinded to the subjects or study personnel.

Permission   Agreement of parents or guardians of a child or ward to participate in clinical research.

Phases of Pharmaceutical Clinical Trials   Clinical trials are often categorized into four general phases. Test articles may be evaluated in two or more phases simultaneously in different trials, and some trials may overlap two phases. *Phase I*—The first stage of testing in humans is to determine safety, duration of action and pharmacologic effect (how the drug is absorbed, distributed, metabolized, and excreted). Subjects are usually healthy volunteers, but may be patients with diseases such as cancer or AIDS. *Phase II*—To demonstrate safety and efficacy, studies are performed on small group of subjects (100–300) with the target disease. *Phase III*—To provide conclusive evidence of safety and effectiveness for a specific indication, studies are performed on a larger subject group (several hundred to several thousand) with the target disease. *Phase IV*—To establish long-term safety and efficacy, studies are performed after FDA approval.

Placebo   An inactive agent given to a study subject instead of an active drug. To keep subjects and investigators unaware of the treatment assignment, the placebo often matches the study drug in appearance. This helps to blind the study and reduces bias based on knowledge of the treatment. Often called a *sugar pill*.

Pre-Clinical Trials   Animal studies that provide safety data and information about an investigational product's activities and effects. Pre-clinical trials provide a framework for clinical trial (human) testing.

Pre-Market Approval (PMA)   A PMA application is submitted to the FDA to request approval to market a device. The FDA evaluates the safety and effectiveness of Class III devices, especially those that support or sustain human life, are of substantial importance in preventing impairment of human health, or that present a potential, unreasonable risk of illness or injury.

Protocol   A document that identifies the plan or set of rules for conducting a specific clinical trial, and states the objectives, design, methodology, statistical considerations, and organization of a trial.

Protocol Amendment   A written description of changes to, or the formal clarification of, a protocol.

Quality Assurance   The planned and systematic actions that are established to ensure that a trial is conducted and data are collected and recorded according to the protocol, standards of good clinical practice, and applicable regulations.

Randomization   The process of assigning trial subjects to treatment and control groups using the element of chance; random treatment assignments are performed to reduce bias.

Risk   The possibility of harm or discomfort for subjects participating in a clinical trial.

Serious Adverse Event (also Serious Adverse Experience) (SAE)   An adverse drug experience occurring at any dose that results in any of the following outcomes: (1) death, (2) a threat to the life of the subject, (3) inpatient hospitalization or prolongation of existing hospitalization, (4) persistent or significant disability/incapacity, or (5) a congenital anomaly/birth defect. Important medical events that may not result in death, be life-threatening, or require hospitalization may be considered a serious adverse experience when, based upon appropriate medical judgment, they may jeopardize the patient and require medical or surgical intervention to prevent one of the outcomes listed above.

Single-Blind Study   See *Blinding*.

Site Coordinator   The individual at the study site who is typically responsible for the day-to-day conduct of study activities, including case report form completion, study file maintenance, investigator assistance, study drug administration, and communicating with the sponsor. Also called *trial coordinator, study coordinator, research coordinator, clinical research coordinator, research nurse*, and *protocol nurse*.

Source Documents   Original documents, data, and records from which patient case report forms are compiled. Source documents include: hospital records, clinic and office charts, laboratory and procedural reports, patient diaries, pharmacy dispensing records, and x-rays.

Source Document Verification   Process of comparing data recorded on patient case report forms with the data originally recorded on source documents.

Sponsor   An individual, company, institution, or organization that initiates a clinical investigation. The sponsor must comply with the responsibilities outlined in the regulations.

Sponsor-Investigator   An individual who both initiates and conducts a clinical trial, and who directs the use, administration, and distribution of the investigational product. The obligations of a sponsor-investigator include both those of the sponsor and the investigator.

Standard Operating Procedure (SOP)   Detailed written instructions that provide a structure to ensure that activities are performed in a consistent manner.

Study-Directed Inspections   Inspections conducted periodically to determine compliance with FDA regulations. Generally, the inspections are conducted for a specific drug, device, biologic, or study as a result of a pending application for marketing approval. Also called *surveillance and routine inspections*.

Sub-Investigator   An individual member of a clinical trial team to whom trial-related activities or procedures have been delegated by the investigator. While some sponsors ask sites to list non-physicians participating in the study in section 6 of the Form FDA 1572, the FDA regards sub-investigators as those individuals authorized by the PI to make medical judgments and decisions regarding study patients.

Subject   An individual who participates in clinical research, either as a recipient of the test article or of the control. A subject may be either a healthy human or a patient.

Unblinding   Determination of the study treatment administered. Unblinding should only occur when subsequent clinical treatment depends upon knowledge of the study treatment given.

Unanticipated Adverse Device Effect   Death, any life-threatening problem, or any serious adverse effect on health or safety caused by or associated with a device if that effect, problem, or death was not previously identified in nature, severity, or degree of incidence in the application. Any other serious problem associated with a device that relates to the rights, safety, or welfare of subjects.

Unexpected Adverse Drug Reaction   An adverse reaction, the nature or severity of which is not consistent with the applicable product information in the investigators' brochure for an unapproved investigational product, or on the package insert/summary of product characteristics for an approved product.

Unexpected Adverse Event   An adverse event that is unexpected for the investigational product and has not been reported in the investigator's brochure or package insert or is an event that is being reported in greater severity or frequency than the same event previously reported.

Vulnerable Subjects   Individuals whose willingness to volunteer in a study may be unduly influenced by expectation of benefits, fear of retaliatory response, or lack of ability to understand trial-related issues. Some groups identified as vulnerable subjects are prisoners, children, unborn fetuses, homeless persons, and those incapable of giving consent.

List of Illustrations

"Somewhere, something incredible is waiting to be known."

—Carl Sagan

"It had become clear to me that medicine could hardly hope to become a science until… qualified men could give themselves to uninterrupted study and investigation. I knew nothing of the cost of research; I did not realize its enormous difficulty; the only thing I saw was the overwhelming and universal need and the infinite promise, world-wide, universal, and eternal."

—*John D. Rockefeller, 1897*

In This Chapter

Milestones in the history of food and drug safety—from the first food laws to the founding of the FDA to the fight over tobacco

Lessons from a Horse Named Jim

A History of Regulations Affecting Clinical Research

The First Clinical Trial?

The Book of Daniel in the Bible describes a comparative trial—in which Daniel experiments with feeding youthful palace servants legumes and porridge rather than the rich meats eaten by the king and his court.

The result?

"And at the end of ten days their countenances appeared fairer and fatter in flesh than all the children which did eat the portion of the king's meat." (Daniel 1:15)

Since early civilizations, people have been concerned about the quality and safety of foods and medicines. The first English food law was enacted in 1202 when King John of England proclaimed the **Assize of Bread**, a law prohibiting the adulteration of bread with such ingredients as ground peas or beans.[1] One of the earliest food and drug laws in United States history was enacted in 1785, when the state of Massachusetts passed the first general food adulteration law.

Since then, many events have raised additional issues and concerns related to food and drug safety. These events have led to regulations that affect the way we investigate and manufacture new products, including medicines and medical devices. The following are only a few of the events and subsequent laws or responses, drawn primarily from American history, that shape and regulate how we conduct clinical research of investigational products in the United States today.

1848 The first United States federal regulation dates back to this year, when American soldiers died as a result of adulterated quinine in the Mexican War. In response to these deaths, Congress passed the **Drug Importation Act**, requiring U.S. Customs inspections to stop the entry of adulterated drugs from overseas.

1901 A horse named Jim was used to prepare an antitoxin for diphtheria. After the death of 13 children who received the antitoxin, authorities discovered that the horse had developed tetanus and therefore contaminated the antitoxin. As a result of this tragedy, Congress passed the **Biologic Control Act of 1902**, giving the government regulatory power over antitoxin and vaccine development. As reported in the *N.Y. Medical Journal*, the horse named Jim "was killed at once."

1906 The original **Food and Drugs Act** was passed by Congress and signed into law by President Theodore Roosevelt, prohibiting interstate commerce in misbranded and adulterated food, drugs, and drinks. This law, authorizing the federal government to monitor food purity and the safety of medicines, was initially enforced by the Bureau of Chemistry.

1931 The Bureau of Chemistry was reorganized in 1927; four years later the group responsible for enforcing the Food and Drugs Act was renamed the **Food and Drug Administration (FDA)**.

1932 The **Tuskegee Study of Untreated Syphilis in the Negro Male** was initiated under the auspices of the U.S. Public Health Service. Subjects included 399 poor black sharecroppers with latent syphilis and 201 men without the disease who served as controls. The men were told that they were being treated for "bad blood" and were not told of the purpose of the study. When penicillin became available in the 1950s, treatment was not offered to the men with syphilis. It was not until 1972, 40 years after this study began, that it became widely known that this study followed the untreated course of syphilis and that subjects were deprived of effective treatment in order not to interrupt the project.

1937 107 people, mostly children, died after taking a medication labeled "elixir of sulfanilamide." It turned out that it was not an elixir (by definition an alcohol solution), but a diethylene glycol (antifreeze) solution. The FDA successfully removed the product from the market, not because it proved fatal, but only because it was mislabeled. This incident emphasized the need for drug safety prior to marketing.

1938 The following year, Congress passed the **Food, Drug, and Cosmetic Act of 1938** which expanded the role of the FDA, requiring predistribution clearance for the *safety* of new drugs, and extended the FDA's control to include cosmetics and devices.

1940–45 Nazi medical personnel conducted medical experiments on unwilling non-German civilians and prisoners-of-war. Abuses of these individuals included sterilization, euthanasia, and exposure to temperature extremes, bacteria, and untested drugs. The Nuremberg War Crime Trials exposed how these experiments were conducted in concentration camps including Auschwitz and Dachau.

1947 During the Nuremberg War Crime Trials, ten standards were drafted as a method for judging the physicians and scientists who had conducted biomedical experiments on concentration camp prisoners. These standards, known as the **Nuremberg Code**, became the prototype for future codes intended to assure that future human research would be conducted in an ethical manner.

1962 Thousands of western European babies were born with birth defects to mothers taking the sedative thalidomide. While never approved for marketing in the U.S., thalidomide was being used extensively in research in American women. Of the 3879 American women of childbearing age who received thalidomide, nine women gave birth to infants with phocomelia, a defective development of the arms and/or legs in which the hands and feet are attached close to the body. Until this time, there was no requirement to notify the FDA about the investigational use of drugs. Therefore, when the FDA approximated the number of U.S. physicians using thalidomide, the FDA's estimate of 40 to 50 fell far short of the well over 1000 physicians actually using the drug in an investigational setting. The magnitude of this tragedy spurred further regulation and a demand that *both efficacy and safety* be demonstrated before marketing. This mandate was incorporated into the **Kefauver-Harris Amendment** to the Food, Drug, and Cosmetic Act.

Also at this time, President John F. Kennedy proclaimed the **Consumer Bill of Rights** in a message to Congress. Included are the right to safety, the right to be informed, the right to choose, and the right to be heard.

1964 At its 18th Medical Assembly held in Helsinki, Finland, the World Medical Association produced a document known as the **Declaration of Helsinki** prefaced with a binding statement for physicians: "The health of my patient will be my first consideration." The declaration, amended by the World Medical Assembly in 1975, 1983, 1989, and again in 1996, provides guidelines for the ethical treatment of human subjects (see Appendix A). The Helsinki declaration provides a clear distinction between situations where a subject benefits from research participation and a situation where benefit is not expected. The basic elements of the declaration are incorporated into the Code of Federal Regulations.

1972 The regulation of biologics—including serums, vaccines, and blood products—was transferred from the National Institutes of Health to the FDA.

1974 The **National Research Act** was signed into law, creating the National Commission for the Protection of Human Subjects of Biomedical and Behavioral Research. This committee was created to identify the basic ethical principles on which clinical research should be based.

1976 The **Medical Device Amendments** to the Food, Drug, and Cosmetic Act provides exemption from pre-market notification, pre-market approval, and other controls of the Food, Drug and Cosmetic Act in order to encourage the discovery and development of useful medical devices.

1979 The National Commission for the Protection of Human Subjects of Biomedical and Behavioral Research issued the **Belmont Report**, a statement of basic ethical principles and guidelines for the protection of human research subjects (see Appendix A). Three basic principles were identified: (1) *respect* for persons, including respect for the decisions of autonomous individuals and protection of those with diminished autonomy, (2) *beneficence*, or an obligation to do no harm, maximizing possible benefits and minimizing possible harm, and (3) *justice*, the fair and equal distribution of clinical research burdens and benefits.

1980–81 The FDA and Department of Health and Human Services incorporated the principles set forth in the Belmont Report into laws regarding clinical research. The basic regulations governing the practice of clinical research for investigational drugs were issued in Title 21 of the **Code of Federal Regulations** *(21 CFR)*. 21 CFR Part 50 (21 CFR § 50) deals with the protection of human subjects, 21 CFR § 56 addresses Institutional Review Boards (IRBs), and 21 CFR § 312 lists regulations pertaining to an Investigational New Drug application, the general responsibilities of investigators, the control of investigational drugs, record keeping and retention, and assurance of IRB reviews. Some components of the CFR were written as early as 1975 and have continued to be revised and amended.

1983 The **Orphan Drug Act** was passed, enabling the FDA to promote research into and approval and marketing of otherwise unprofitable drugs needed for treating rare diseases.

1988 The **Food and Drug Administration Act** made the FDA an agency of the Department of Health and Human Services with a Commissioner of Food and Drugs appointed by the President.

1990 Congress passed the **Safe Medical Devices Act**, requiring medical device users such as hospitals and nursing homes to report promptly to the FDA any incidents that reasonably suggest that a medical device caused or contributed to the death, serious illness, or injury of a patient. Device users were also required to establish methods for tracing and locating patients depending on such devices.

1990 The movement toward developing standard international guidelines and regulations began when representatives from Europe, Japan, and the United States met at the **International Conference on Harmonization** *of Technical Requirements for Registration of Pharmaceuticals for Human Use (ICH)*. A committee was formed to make recommendations for greater standardization in clinical research, with the goal of reducing or eliminating duplication of testing in various countries. The objective of this effort is better use of human, animal, and material resources. A secondary aim is the elimination of delays in global drug development while maintaining safeguards on quality, safety, efficacy, and regulatory obligations to protect public health.

1991 The FDA published regulations to accelerate the review of drugs for life-threatening diseases.

1995 The FDA declared cigarettes to be "drug delivery devices" and proposed restrictions on marketing and sales to reduce smoking by young people.

1997 The **Food and Drug Administration Modernization Act** reauthorized the Prescription Drug User Fee Act of 1992 and mandated the most wide-ranging reforms in agency practices since 1938. Provisions include measures to accelerate review of devices, advertising unapproved uses of approved drugs and devices, health claims for foods in agreement with published data by a reputable public health source, and development of good guidance practices for agency decision-making.

2000 In response to the 1999 death of an 18-year-old subject who died from multiple-organ failure brought on by the infusion of genetically altered cold viruses into his diseased liver, the FDA and NIH took a number of steps to ensure patient protection and fully informed consent in gene therapy trials. Apparently subjects in the gene therapy trial, including the one who died, were not informed that monkeys had died from the therapy before it was given to humans, and that several previous participants had suffered serious toxic reactions to the kind of treatment being given.

One of the steps taken was to rename and transfer the **Office for Human Research Protections (OHRP)**, formerly called the Office for Protection from Research Risks (OPRR), from the NIH to the Office of the Assistant Secretary of the Department of Health and Human Services (HHS). This organizational change expanded its role and elevated its stature and effectiveness, placing even stronger emphasis on the protection of human subjects.

This overview of the historical events affecting the regulation of clinical research reveals only a short period of time since the implementation of laws governing clinical research and the protection of human subjects. Many of the changes in regulations have been in response to isolated and often catastrophic events rather than based on a prospective plan. The face of clinical research and the conduct of trials will undoubtedly continue to change as new events unfold and shape the future of this field.

References

1 *http://www.fda.gov/opacom/backgrounders/miles.html* FDA Backgrounder: Milestones in U.S. Food and Drug Law History

"Experience is fallacious and judgement difficult."

—Hippocrates

The Process

Developing New Drugs and Devices

The Drug Development Process

Developing new drug treatments is often an expensive and lengthy process, with an average time from pre-clinical studies through FDA approval of nine years or more, and costing up to an estimated half a billion dollars. Many compounds never make it out of the laboratory, many drugs fail animal testing, and still others demonstrate toxicity or a lack of efficacy in human studies, leaving only a small percentage of new drugs that reach the market. In 1998, while there were approximately 11,000 compounds in various stages of testing by pharmaceutical and biotechnology companies, the FDA took 199 actions, 90 of which were approvals, on original New Drug Applications. This number was similar in 1999 when the FDA took 190

New Drug Development Timeline[1]

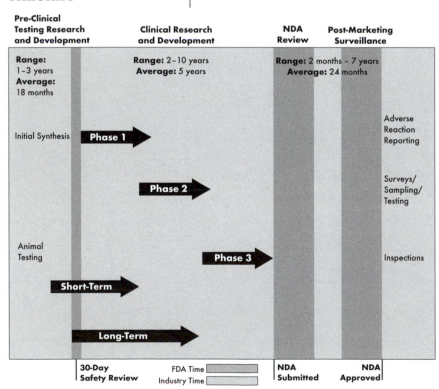

Pre-Clinical Testing Research and Development	Clinical Research and Development	NDA Review	Post-Marketing Surveillance
Range: 1–3 years **Average:** 18 months	**Range:** 2–10 years **Average:** 5 years	**Range:** 2 months – 7 years **Average:** 24 months	

Initial Synthesis — Phase 1

Phase 2

Adverse Reaction Reporting

Surveys/ Sampling/ Testing

Animal Testing — Phase 3 — Inspections

Short-Term

Long-Term

30-Day Safety Review

FDA Time
Industry Time

NDA Submitted

NDA Approved

actions on original New Drug Applications, 83 of which were approvals.[2]

The approval process in the United States is rigorous, providing the opportunity to carefully evaluate the treatment under investigation. The FDA oversees and monitors the process, setting the appropriate regulations and guidelines to ensure that only safe and effective products reach the public. To accomplish this, the FDA requires the sponsors of new treatments to conduct studies in a carefully prescribed manner.

Pre-Clinical Studies

When new compounds show potential in laboratory tests, studies are designed to evaluate these compounds for potential pharmacologic use. These studies of a new compound or drug, generally performed in animals, are referred to as "pre-clinical" studies. Pre-clinical studies help establish boundaries for the safe use of the treatment when human testing begins. Special care is taken to evaluate the possibility of long-term, adverse effects such as the onset of cancer, interference with reproduction, or the induction of birth defects. Many new drugs and treatments are abandoned during pre-clinical studies, having proven to be unsafe in animals. When sufficient data are obtained to warrant study in human subjects, the sponsor of the new product must submit an application to the FDA requesting permission to initiate clinical trials.

The Investigational New Drug (IND) Application

The application to request permission to begin human testing is commonly referred to as an Investigational New Drug (IND) application, actually a shortened version of the official title of *Notice of Claimed Investigational Exemption for a New Drug*. An IND is not an application for approval,

One of Medicine's Most Celebrated Clinical Trials

Louis Pasteur treated patients exposed to rabies with an experimental anti-rabies vaccine. All the treated patients survived. Since untreated rabies was 100% fatal, it was easy to conclude that the vaccine was effective.

Some (but not all) of the Required Components of an IND

- A completed Form FDA 1571 *Investigational New Drug* application that serves as the cover sheet (see Appendix F)

- An introductory statement and general description of the plan for studying the treatment

- An investigator's brochure containing information pertaining to the investigational drug formulation, pharmacokinetics, toxicology, safety and effectiveness from previous studies, and potential anticipated risks and side effects based on prior experience

- A protocol for each planned study

- A summary of previous human experience with the drug, including information acquired if the drug was investigated or marketed in another country, or if the drug was used in combination with other drugs previously investigated or marketed

A complete listing of the required IND content and format can be found in the Code of Federal Regulations, 21 CFR § 312.23. Protocols are discussed in greater detail in Chapter 5.

Clinical Holds

Reasons the FDA might issue a clinical hold include:

- Exposure of human subjects to unreasonable risks

- Lack of qualifications of the clinical investigators named in the IND in terms of their training and/or experience

- An incomplete or erroneous investigator's brochure

- Deficient design of the plan or protocol in meeting its objectives

but rather an application for exemption from the laws that normally prevent the distribution and use of pharmaceutical agents that have not been FDA-approved. The IND allows the use of an investigational agent in human subjects for the sole purpose of conducting clinical trials.

Once an Investigational New Drug application is received, the FDA typically has 30 days to notify the sponsor if a "clinical hold," a delay or suspension of the proposed investigations identified in the IND, is being issued. A complete listing of the grounds for imposing a clinical hold can be found in the Code of Federal Regulations, 21 CFR § 312.42 (b).

If the FDA does not respond with questions or issue a clinical hold within 30 days of the date the initial IND application was received, the sponsor may proceed with the planned studies.

Clinical Trial Phases

The studies performed under an Investigational New Drug application are often classified into phases as if they are separate and distinct steps in the process. However, in reality the phases overlap and trials in one phase are often conducted simultaneously with trials in other phases. In general, clinical trials are classified into the following phases.[3]

Phase I: Evaluation of Clinical Pharmacology and Toxicity

The first phase of testing is aimed at determining a safe dose range in which a drug can be administered, the method of absorption and distribution in the body, and possible toxicity. A primary consideration in Phase I trials is limitation of risk to the subjects.

Phase I trials:

- are conducted to determine the appropriate dose range with regard to safety and toxicity (not to evaluate efficacy);
- are conducted in a limited number (usually 20–80) of healthy volunteers or patients (such as patients with cancer or AIDS);
- often take 9–18 months to complete.

Many compounds are abandoned in Phase I testing because of problems with safety or toxicity.

Phase II: Initial Evaluation for Safety and Treatment Effect

Once safety and dosage have been determined in Phase I trials, small-scale, well-controlled Phase II trials evaluate preliminary safety and efficacy in the targeted population. The safety of subjects is still a primary consideration.

Phase II trials:

- are conducted in a relatively limited number (usually 100–300) of patients who have the disease or condition to be treated;
- often involve hospitalized patients who can be closely monitored;
- may focus on dose-response, dosing schedule, or other issues related to preliminary safety and efficacy;
- often take 1–3 years to complete.

Additional animal testing may also be done simultaneously to obtain long-term safety information. If studies show that the new drug is safe and useful, testing may proceed to Phase III trials.

Phase III: Large-Scale Treatment Evaluation

Phase III trials involve the most extensive testing to fully assess safety, efficacy, and drug dosage in a large group of patients with the specific disease to be treated.

Clinical Trial Phases

Phase I:
First stage of testing in humans

Phase II:
Preliminary safety and efficacy studies

Phase III:
Expanded large-scale studies

Phase IV:
Post-marketing studies

2. The Process: Developing New Drugs and Devices

Phase III trials:

- are conducted in larger (several hundred to several thousand) and more diverse patient groups for whom the drug is ultimately intended;
- make comparisons between the new treatment and standard therapy or placebo;
- study a drug used by practicing physicians in the same manner as it would be used after marketing;
- often take 2–5 years to complete.

Phase III studies often produce much of the information that is eventually used for package labeling and the package insert.

The phases of trials may be further classified into subsets of phases. For example, Phase II trials may be divided into Phase IIa and IIb. *Phase IIa studies* are pilot trials to evaluate efficacy and safety in selected populations with the disease or condition while *Phase IIb studies* are well-controlled trials to evaluate efficacy and safety, usually the most rigorous demonstration of a medicine's safety, and sometimes referred to as pivotal trials.[4] *Phase IIIb studies* are trials conducted after a New Drug Application has been submitted to the FDA but before approval and marketing. Phase IIIb trials may supplement earlier trials or may obtain additional information, such as quality of life or economic information.

New Drug Application (NDA)

Once the proposed clinical studies are completed and analyzed, and the sponsor believes adequate positive information has been obtained to request marketing approval, the sponsor submits a New Drug Application (NDA) to the FDA. The NDA contains extensive data on the investigational agent, results of the clinical trials conducted, and safety data, and may include copies of individual case report forms. Once received, the New Drug Application is given to the group of FDA reviewers responsible for that drug classification. Complete requirements for an NDA submission can be found in 21 CFR § 312.

FDA Review Groups

As the principal agency responsible for the safety and efficacy of pharmaceutical agents, biological products, and medical devices produced in the United States, the FDA reviews the clinical research performed and assesses the product's risks, weighing them against the benefits.

CDER and CBER

The groups within the FDA who hold the primary responsibility to review and approve or disapprove new drugs and biologics are:

1 *Center for Drug Evaluation and Research (CDER)* — responsible for both prescription and over-the-counter drugs. CDER requires new drugs to be both safe and effective and makes a determination of whether the new drug produces the proclaimed benefits without causing side effects that would outweigh the benefits.

2 *Center for Biologics Evaluation and Research (CBER)* — responsible for blood and blood products, vaccines, allergenics, and biologics (medical preparations made from living organisms and their products). CBER examines blood bank operations and ensures the purity and effectiveness of biological products such as insulin. CBER's regulation of biological products has expanded in recent years to include a wide variety of new products, including gene therapy, banked human tissues, and xenotransplantation.

In addition to the FDA review groups, outside reviewers contribute to the review process as members of FDA Advisory Committees. The primary roles of the advisory committees are to provide independent expert scientific advice and to help the FDA make sound decisions about

Brave New World

Recent work in the area of recombinant DNA and gene transfer as well as xenotransplantation has created potential new therapies that are classified as biological products.

Gene transfer trials target a number of diseases, including cancer, HIV infection, cystic fibrosis, and hemophilia. The primary assumption behind gene therapy is that inserting normal genes into the DNA of the cells containing malfunctioning genes may cause the cells to function properly, and may either reduce or eliminate the symptoms of the disease. For example, gene therapy might be used in a person with hemophilia, which is caused by the malfunctioning of the gene that makes the clotting factor. If gene therapy is successful, a person with hemophilia would be able to make their own clotting factor after receiving gene therapy, instead of requiring repeated treatments with clotting factor.[5]

Xenotransplantation involves the "use of live cells, tissues, or organs from a nonhuman animal source transplanted or implanted into a human, or used for ex vivo contact with human body fluids, cells, tissues or organs that are subsequently given to a human recipient."[6] Because of the continued shortage of donated human organs as well as advances in the areas of immunology and tissue rejection, xenotransplantation is of increasing interest and may hold the potential for treating a wide range of disorders. However, xenotransplantation also holds the risk of transmitting infectious agents from animal donors to the human recipients as well as to humans in close contact with recipients. For this reason, scientific and agency review is critical to assure the safety of human subjects as well as the public at large.

Note: Biological products, drugs, and medical devices sourced from nonliving animal cells, tissues, or organs (for example, porcine insulin and porcine heart valves) are not considered xenotransplantation products.

product approval. Advisory committees make recommendations but the FDA makes the final decisions.

In 1999, the median time required by the FDA to review and approve New Drug Applications was just under 12 months. The FDA also has an expedited review process for "priority drugs," those that represent an advance in medical treatment. The median review time for the 28 priority drugs approved in 1999 was just over 6 months.

Treatment Use of Investigational Drugs

A drug that is not approved for marketing may be under clinical investigation for a serious or life-threatening illness in patients for whom there is no comparable or satisfactory alternative. In such cases, a treatment IND may be issued for the purpose of making promising new drugs available to desperately ill patients as early in the drug development process as possible, before the drug is marketed.[7] A treatment IND may be issued after there are enough data to indicate that the investigational agent "may be effective" and does not have unreasonable risks. Because safety and side-effect data are collected, information obtained under treatment INDs also contributes to the body of knowledge about the agent.[8]

Compassionate Use of Investigational Drugs

There are occasions when a clinical trial has ended and patient(s) are allowed to continue taking the investigational drug, benefiting from its use while the sponsor pursues marketing approval.[9] This may be referred to as "compassionate" use of an investigational drug.

Compassionate use of a drug may also be granted when a drug that has been marketed or is under investigation in another country (but not available in the U.S.) is the only reasonable and available treatment. Compassionate use has also been approved in cases where a patient does not meet a clinical trial's eligibility criteria, but the drug has the possibility of benefit to the patient, and there is no other treatment available.

Emergency Use of Investigational Drugs

There are times when the need for an investigational drug may arise in an emergency situation in which there isn't adequate time to submit an IND. In such a case, the FDA may authorize shipment of the drug for a specific use before an IND is submitted. This authorization is given with the condition that the sponsor submit an IND as soon as possible after receiving FDA authorization.[10]

"Orphan" Drugs

Orphan products are defined as drugs used to treat diseases or conditions affecting less than 200,000 persons in the United States. In reality, most of these conditions occur in far fewer patients than this, with almost half of the conditions on the orphan drug list affecting 25,000 or fewer people. These small patient populations make it difficult for a sponsor to profit from the marketing of the

Defibrotide, a drug under investigation in Italy, has anti-thrombotic, anti-ischemic, anti-inflammatory, and thrombolytic properties. The compassionate use of defibrotide has recently been allowed in the U.S. for the treatment of a patient with severe hepatic veno-occlusive disease.

1999 Drug Review Accomplishments by the FDA:

- 83 new drugs
- 35 new molecular entities
- 97 new uses for already approved drugs
- 4 over-the-counter drugs
- 4 new uses for an over-the-counter drug
- 186 generic equivalents for prescription and over-the-counter drugs
- 43 first-ever generic approvals
- 16 orphan uses

Priority drugs approved in 1999 include a drug (epirubicin hydrochloride) to treat early-stage breast cancer that has spread to the lymph nodes under the arm and has been treated surgically, a short-term treatment (caffeine citrate) for apnea in children, a new protease inhibitor (amprenavir) for use in children as young as 4 and in adults in combination with other anti-retrovirals for HIV infection, and the first drug (sirolimus) in a new class of immunosuppressant agents that prevent organ rejection in people with transplants.[11]

19

drug, so there has been little incentive for pharmaceutical companies to develop products in these areas.

To reverse the trend of avoiding orphan drug development, Congress passed the *Orphan Drug Act of 1983* granting special privileges and marketing incentives. The passage of this act gave research groups and drug companies financial incentives to develop and adopt orphan drugs and—equally importantly—focused public, government, and industry attention on the plight of those who suffer from rare diseases. The act provides grant money to support the development of orphan drugs, allows for FDA support in protocol development, provides tax credits, and gives the sponsor of an orphan drug legal protection against the introduction of an identical competing product for seven years.[12]

Developing New Devices

There are similarities between the drug development process and the device development process, including the fact that both are governed by the same informed consent and IRB regulations (21 CFR § 50 and 56). There are, however, many differences in the process and other applicable regulations.

What is a Medical Device?

A medical device is defined, in part, as any health care product that does not achieve its primary intended purposes by chemical action or by being metabolized. Medical devices include products such as surgical lasers, wheelchairs, sutures, pacemakers, vascular grafts, intraocular lenses, and orthopedic pins.[13]

Classes of Medical Devices

Products that meet the definition of a medical device are assigned to one of three regulatory classes based on the level of risk to users/patients, and therefore the level of control and FDA oversight necessary to assure the safety and efficacy of the device as labeled.

General Controls

General controls are the baseline requirements that apply to all medical devices. Unless specifically exempted in the regulations, the general controls require medical devices to be properly labeled and packaged, be cleared for marketing by the FDA (Pre-Market Notification), meet their labeling claims, be designed and manufactured under Good

A medical device is "an instrument, apparatus, implement, machine, contrivance, implant, in vitro reagent, or other similar or related article, including a component part or accessory, which is:

- recognized in the official National Formulary, or the United States Pharmacopoeia, or any supplement to them;

- intended for use in the diagnosis of disease or other conditions, or in the cure, mitigation, treatment, or prevention of disease, in man or other animals; or

- intended to affect the structure or any function of the body of man or other animals, and which does not achieve any of its primary intended purposes through chemical action within or on the body of man or other animals, and which is not dependent upon being metabolized for the achievement of any of its primary intended purposes."[14]

Class of Device		Regulatory Controls	Examples
Class I:	Not life-supporting or life-sustaining; not intended for use that is of substantial importance in preventing impairment of health; does not present potential un-reasonable risk of illness or injury	■ General Controls	■ Crutches, ■ Adhesive bandages
Class II:	Reasonable assurance of safety and effectiveness can be obtained by applying "special controls"	■ General Controls ■ Special Controls	■ Wheelchairs ■ Tampons
Class III:	Insufficient information to show that either Class I or II controls can provide reasonable assurance of safety or effectiveness; includes life-sustaining and life-supporting devices, devices of substantial importance in preventing health impairment, and devices that present a potentially unreasonable risk of illness or injury	■ General Controls ■ Special Controls ■ Pre-Market Approval	■ Heart valves made of new materials ■ Pacemakers ■ Respiratory assist devices ■ Heart assist devices

Manufacturing Practice (21 CFR § 820), and comply with registration, listing, and reporting regulations.

Special Controls

In addition to general controls, Class II devices are subject to special controls, such as special labeling requirements, mandatory performance standards, patient registries, and postmarket surveillance.

Marketing New Devices

Except for certain low risk devices, manufacturers wanting to market a new device must submit a Pre-Market Notification to the FDA. The FDA reviews the notification to determine if the new device is "substantially equivalent" to a device that was marketed before the Medical Device Amendments of 1976 (i.e., a pre-amendment or predicate device). If the new device is deemed substantially equivalent to a pre-amendment device, it may be marketed immediately and is regulated in the same regulatory class as the pre-amendment device to which it is equivalent. Many devices are cleared for commercial distribution in the U.S. by this process.

Substantial Equivalence

Substantial equivalence means that when compared to the predicate device, the new device:

■ has the same intended use, *and* has the same technological characteristics,

or

■ has different technological characteristics that do not raise new safety and effectiveness questions, assuming the sponsor demonstrates that the new device is as safe and effective as the predicate device.

A device cannot be marketed in the U.S. until the applicant receives an order from the FDA declaring a device to be substantially equivalent. However, if the device is deemed not to be substantially equivalent, it must undergo clinical testing and pre-market approval before it can be marketed (unless reclassified into a lower regulatory class).

Pre-Market Approval

Pre-Market Approval (PMA) is similar to the New Drug Application (NDA) that is required before marketing new drugs. PMA, an application submitted to the FDA to request approval to market a device, evaluates the safety and effectiveness of Class III devices; however, not all Class III devices require an approved PMA to be marketed.

Unlike Pre-Market Notification, approval of a PMA is given when the FDA determines there is evidence supporting reasonable assurance that the device is safe and effective for its intended use. The process of obtaining Pre-Market Approval starts with an Investigational Device Exemption (IDE), similar to the IND for drugs, and the goal is to establish the safety and effectiveness of the device.

All clinical investigations of medical devices must comply with the same informed consent and IRB regulations that govern investigations of drugs and biologics (21 CFR § 50 and 56). The current regulations regarding medical device investigations, enacted as part of the Medical Device Amendments of 1976 and the Safe Medical Devices Act of 1990, may be found in 21 CFR § 800–1299. These regulations include Pre-Market Notification found in 21 CFR § 807, Subpart E, Investigational Device Exemption (IDE) requirements found in 21 CFR § 812, Pre-Market Approval (PMA) regulations in 21 CFR § 814, and Quality System Regulations (QSR) found in 21 CFR § 820.

Substantially Equivalent Devices

Devices determined by the FDA to be "substantially equivalent" are often referred to as 510(k) devices. Pre-Market Notification [510(k)] must be submitted for Class I, Class II, and some Class III devices at least 90 days before marketing unless the device is exempt from 510(k) requirements.

Investigational Device Exemption (IDE) Application

Similar to an Investigational New Drug (IND) application for drugs, the Investigational Device Exemption (IDE) application allows manufacturers to ship and use unapproved medical devices intended solely for investigational use in human subjects. IDE regulations apply to most, but not all, clinical studies performed in the U.S. that are undertaken to collect safety and effectiveness data about an investigational medical device. An investigational device is one that has not been given 510(k) clearance or pre-market approval, but is exempted from these requirements in order to collect the safety and effectiveness data needed. Investigational use also includes evaluation of device modifications and new uses of an approved device.

Risk Assessment

Based on the assessment of risk to users, devices are either categorized as "significant risk devices" and subject to full IDE regulations, or categorized as "non-significant risk devices" and subject to abbreviated IDE regulations. The initial risk assessment is made by the sponsor (usually the device manufacturer) and should be based on the proposed use of the device in the investigation.

A *significant risk device* is one that presents a potential for serious risk to the health, safety, or welfare of a subject, and meets one of the criteria found in 21 CFR § 812 Section 3(m), such as an implant or a device that is life-supporting or life-sustaining. Both FDA and IRB review and approval are required before the investigation may begin at a site.

A *non-significant risk device* is one that does not pose a significant risk to subjects and does not meet the above definition for significant risk. Non-significant risk device studies have fewer regulatory controls than significant risk studies and are governed by abbreviated requirements in 21 CFR § 812.2 (b), but must comply with the same IRB and informed consent regulations. Some of the differences in the regulations are in the approval process, record keeping, and reporting requirements. The non-significant risk category of devices was created to avoid delay and expense when the anticipated risks did not justify FDA involvement.

When a sponsor considers a study to be non-significant risk (NSR), the sponsor provides the reviewing IRB with an explanation of its rationale and seeks approval for an NSR study of the device. The IRB may ask the sponsor for additional information and may agree or disagree with the sponsor's assessment. If the IRB agrees with the NSR assessment and approves the study, no FDA submission or review is necessary before human studies begin. If the IRB disagrees with the NSR assessment, the sponsor must notify the FDA that a significant risk (SR) assessment has been made, and must submit an IDE application before starting clinical trials.

There is no requirement to report the start of an NSR study to the FDA; however, the requirements for IRB review, informed consent, adverse event reporting, and labeling do apply. Therefore, when an NSR study is being conducted, the IRB is, in a sense, serving as the FDA's surrogate. Sponsors may want to voluntarily seek advice from or inform the FDA about proceeding with the study without filing an IDE, since the FDA has the authority to later disagree with the NSR assessment.

	Significant Risk (SR) Device Study	Non-Significant Risk (NSR) Device Study
FDA approval before starting study	X	
IRB approval before starting study	X	X
Informed consent	X	X
IDE application submitted to the FDA	X	

25

Significant Risk Devices	Non-significant Risk Devices
Extended wear contact lenses	Daily wear contact lenses
Catheters introduced into the fallopian tubes	Conventional laparoscopes
Collagen implant material for dental application	Dental filling materials
Implantable defibrillator	Externally worn monitors for insulin reactions
Urological catheter with anti-infective coating	General urological catheters
Contraceptive devices (e.g., cervical caps, IUDs, diaphragms, tubal occlusion devices)	Menstrual pads and tampons
Gas machines for anesthesia or analgesia	Transcutaneous electric nerve stimulation devices for treatment of pain
Tissue adhesives for use in surgical applications	Wound dressing, excluding absorbable hemostatic devices and dressings

To assist sponsors and IRBs in the determination of risk, the FDA provides examples of devices in each category. The lists on this page include examples of non-significant risk and significant risk devices. For a more comprehensive list, refer to the Information Sheets about medical devices (www.fda.gov/oc/oha/IRB/toc8.html) and the CDRH website (www.fda.gov/cdrh).

Exempt Studies (or Exempted Investigations)

Certain clinical investigations of devices may be exempt from the full IDE requirements (for SR device studies) or abbreviated IDE requirements (for NSR device studies). The categories of devices for human use that are exempted from the full IDE regulations can be found in 21 CFR § 812.2 and include devices undergoing consumer preference testing and devices intended solely for veterinary use.

Humanitarian Use Device

A humanitarian use device is one that is intended to benefit patients by treating or diagnosing a disease or condition that affects fewer than 4000 individuals in the U.S. per year. The regulations provide for the submission of a Humanitarian Device Exemption (HDE) application, which is similar in form and content to a Pre-Market Approval (PMA) application, but is exempt from a PMA's requirements for effectiveness.[15]

FDA Review Group

Review of medical devices is primarily performed by the *Center for Devices and Radiologic Health* (CDRH) within the FDA. The CDRH is responsible for developing and implementing programs to protect public health in the areas of medical devices and radiologic health. CDRH protects the public health by providing reasonable assurance of the safety and effectiveness of medical devices and by eliminating unnecessary human exposure to radiation emitted from electronic products.

Post-Marketing Surveillance of Drugs and Devices

Once a treatment has FDA approval for marketing, the sponsor must continue to report information about the approved product to the FDA. Health care providers report new findings and/or adverse events about marketed products through two methods:

1 in the context of a Phase IV post-marketing study, or

2 by direct reporting to the product manufacturer or the FDA based on the observation of patients receiving the treatment.

Post-Marketing Drug Studies

Once a drug treatment has been marketed, additional information may be collected by performing Phase IV trials. These trials may be conducted to provide additional information such as testing new dosages, evaluating delayed versus sustained-release formulations, or studying patient subgroups, such as minorities, women, or children. Phase IV studies can further establish the safety and efficacy of the drug and thereby gain greater market acceptability for the product.

Post-Marketing Device Studies

The collection of certain outcome and adverse event data on a device after it is marketed falls in this category. Post-marketing data collection is sometimes required by the FDA, but at other times is done at the discretion of the sponsor.

The **Safe Medical Devices Act of 1990** requires post-marketing surveillance studies on all devices marketed after January 1, 1991, that:

1 are permanent implants, the failure of which may cause serious, adverse health consequences or death;

2 are life-supporting or life-sustaining; or

3 may pose a serious risk to human health.[16]

Post-marketing surveillance is intended primarily to study the performance of a device as used in its target population and to serve as a warning system for detecting potential problems. Manufacturers will receive notice that a medical device is subject to post-marketing surveillance upon 510(k) or PMA acceptance, and must submit a protocol to the FDA within 30 days of introducing the device into interstate commerce.

Direct Reporting Based on Observations

While the FDA is responsible for assuring the safety and efficacy of all regulated marketed drugs, biologics, devices, and nutritional products, health care professionals who monitor patients and report adverse events and product problems are integral to this process. MedWatch, the FDA Medical Products Reporting Program, has been established to educate health professionals about the critical importance of monitoring and reporting events and problems as well as to rapidly communicate new safety information to the medical community. The purpose of MedWatch is to enhance the effectiveness of post-marketing surveillance of medical products used in clinical practice and to rapidly identify significant product-associated health hazards.[17]

Historically, serious adverse events and product problems have been significantly under-reported. This is most likely due to the challenges of determining whether an event is expected or unexpected in the progression of a disease, and determining whether the medical product caused or was coincidental to the event or problem. To improve reporting, MedWatch has clarified events and problems that should be reported and simplified reporting through the use of a single reporting system for health professionals.

Serious adverse events and product problems should be reported to the FDA, either directly or via the product manufacturer, as appropriate. Specifically, within a user facility (hospital, nursing home, etc.), reporting of deaths and serious injuries that occur with the use of devices is mandatory, while the reporting of adverse events and problems with drugs, biologics, and nutritional products is strictly voluntary. However, voluntary reporting by health professionals is vital to the successful and comprehensive post-marketing surveillance of medical products.

MedWatch Form 3500

FDA Form 3500 is the form designed for **voluntary** reporting of adverse events and product problems by health care professionals. When physicians and other health care providers become aware of serious adverse

MedWatch Form 3500

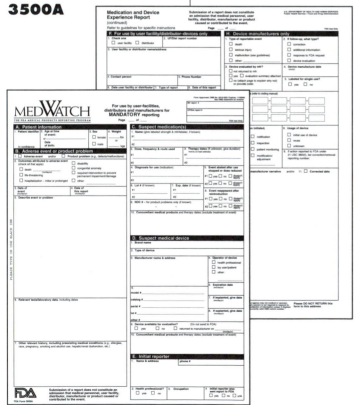

events and product problems in patients outside the setting of a study, the events should be reported either to the product manufacturer, or to the FDA using the MedWatch Form 3500. This form can be used to report experiences with medications, medical devices, special nutritional products, and other FDA-regulated products. Form 3500 may be submitted to the FDA by mail, telephone, fax, or by use of the Internet, although if the product reaction is dangerous or life-threatening, the report should be made by telephone.

MedWatch Form 3500A

MedWatch Form 3500A

FDA Form 3500A is the form designed for the **mandatory** reporting of adverse events and product problems by medical product manufacturers, packers, distributors, and user facilities. Manufacturers and user facilities are required to report deaths and serious injuries that have or may have been caused by (or contributed to) the use of a medical product.

The FDA recognizes that the privacy of patients and of those who report serious adverse events and product problems is an important concern, and actively works to protect confidentiality. Information about reporting requirements and MedWatch forms may be found at http://www.fda.gov/medwatch/index.html.

References

1 http://www.fda.gov/fda/graphics/newdrugspecial/drugchart.pdf

2 CDER 1998 Report to the Nation

3 21 CFR § 312.21 Phases of an investigation

4 Spilker, Bert, Guide to Clinical Trials 1991, page xxii

5 http://www4.od.nih.gov/oba/cover.htm

6 http://www4.od.nih.gov/oba/aboutxeno.htm

7 21 CFR § 312.34 (a) Treatment use of an investigational new drug

8 FDA Information Sheet: Treatment Use of Investigational Drugs, October 1, 1995

9 FDA Information Sheet: Treatment Use of Investigational Drugs, October 1, 1995

10 21 CFR § 312.36 Emergency use of an investigational new drug

11 CDER 1999 Report to the Nation

12 http://www.fda.gov/fdac/special/newdrug/orphan.html Orphan products: New Hope for People with Rare Disorders

13 FDA Information Sheet: Guidance for Institutional Review Boards and Clinical Investigators, 1998 Update, Medical Devices

14 *http://www.fda.gov/cdrh/devadvice/312.html#link_2*

15 *www.fda.gov/cdrh/newdevice.html*

16 U.S. Congress, Safe Medical Device Amendments to the Food, Drug & Cosmetic Act, Section 522(a)(1)(1990)

17 *http://www.fda.gov/medwatch/what.htm*

"In dwelling upon the vital importance of *sound* observation, it must never be lost sight of what observation is for. It is not for the sake of piling up miscellaneous information or curious facts, but for the sake of saving life and increasing health and comfort."

—*Florence Nightingale*

Good Clinical Practice and the Regulations

The regulations quoted in this chapter are current as of the date of this printing. Refer directly to the Code of Federal Regulations, the Federal Register, and FDA Guidance Documents and Information Sheets to obtain the most recent regulatory information.

Good Clinical Practice

Good Clinical Practice (GCP) is the broad term that refers to the accepted standards for conducting clinical research studies. These standards apply to all aspects of clinical trials, from protocol design, monitoring, and auditing, to recording, analysis, and reporting of research data. GCP recognizes the importance of the processes used to conduct research studies, rather than placing value only on the results of the studies.

GCP includes:

1 regulations that are enforceable by law;

2 guidelines that are part of the generally accepted practice although not enforceable by law; and

3 local laws that affect a specific region, city, or state.

Regulations

Federal regulations date back to 1906, when the *Food and Drugs Act* was passed by Congress, authorizing the U.S. government to oversee the safety of drugs. Subsequent regulations pertaining to clinical research were developed in response to a general consensus that research in humans should be ethical and based on the principles set forth in documents such as the Declaration of Helsinki (1964) and the Belmont Report (1979).

Regulations that govern the conduct of clinical trials are published in the Code of Federal Regulations. In addition to regulations for the protection of people participating in clinical research, the Code of Federal Regulations also includes regulations for laboratories (Good Laboratory Practice) and manufacturers (Good Manufacturing Practice) involved in clinical research. As the regulatory

GCP

Good Clinical Practice

A general term referring to the standards of how clinical trials should be conducted including:

■ Regulations

■ Guidelines

■ Local laws

agency responsible for the safety and effectiveness of drugs, biological products, and devices, the FDA oversees the clinical research process and ensures that the regulations are met.

Code of Federal Regulations (CFR)

The laws regulating departments and agencies within the United States government are published in the Code of Federal Regulations (CFR). These regulations are issued by various executive departments and agencies and are divided into 50 "Titles," each assigned to a specific agency and covering subjects ranging from agriculture and banking to clinical research, internal revenue, and wildlife. The titles containing the regulations that apply to clinical research are *Title 21, Food and Drugs*, assigned to the Food and Drug Administration and *Title 45, Public Welfare*, assigned to the National Institutes of Health.

CFR titles have been divided into chapters under the name of the issuing agency. For example, Title 21, Chapter 1 contains regulations issued by the Food and Drug Administration. Each chapter is subsequently subdivided into "Parts" and "Subparts," for example, Title 21, Chapter 1, Part 312 is "Investigational New Drug Application" and Title 21, Chapter 1, Part 312, Subpart D is "Responsibilities of Sponsors and Investigators."

Code of Federal Regulations

- A system to codify (classify) the final rules/regulations published in the Federal Register

- Arranged under 50 titles and further subdivided into chapters, parts, and subparts

- Enforceable by U.S. law

Title 21: Food and Drugs
Food and Drug Administration

Part 11:
Electronic Records; Electronic Signatures

Part 50:
Protection of Human Subjects
Subpart B—Informed Consent of Human Subjects
Subpart D—Additional Safeguards for Children in Clinical Investigations (interim rule)

Part 54:
Financial Disclosure by Clinical Investigators

Part 56:
Institutional Review Boards

Part 58:
Good Laboratory Practice (GLP)

Parts 210–211:
Good Manufacturing Practices (GMP)

Part 312:
Investigational New Drug (IND) Application
Subpart D—Responsibilities of Sponsors and Investigators

Part 314:
New Drug Application (NDA)

Part 600–680:
Biologic Products

Part 812:
Investigational Device Exemption (IDE)

Part 814:
Pre-Market Approval of Medical Devices

Part 820:
Quality System Regulation

Title 45: Public Welfare
National Institutes of Health

Part 46:
Protection of Human Subjects
Subpart B—Additional Protections Pertaining to Research Involving Fetuses, Pregnant Women, and Human in Vitro Fertilization
Subpart C—Additional Protections Involving Prisoners as Subjects
Subpart D—Additional Protections for Children Involved as Subjects in Research

The FDA operates under Title 21 in the oversight of clinical trials of investigational drugs, biologic products, or medical devices. These regulations also apply to clinical trials investigating new indications for a previously marketed product. When clinical trials involve federal funding, such as trials conducted by the National Institutes of Health (NIH) or the Centers for Disease Control and Prevention (CDC), *Title 45, Public Welfare*, becomes applicable as well. It is important to determine which regulations are in effect for each specific trial. While many federally funded trials fall under both Title 21 and 45 (when an investigational drug, biologic, or device is involved), some federally funded trials fall only under Title 45. One example of a trial that must meet Title 45 regulations but does not require FDA oversight would be an NIH-funded trial comparing two marketed products in a patient population consistent with the product labeling.

While the CFR contains the minimum requirements for the conduct of clinical research in the United States, local governments (state, county), study sponsors, and IRBs often have additional requirements. It is important to note the difference between those required by the federal and local governments, since they apply to all trials conducted at a specific site, versus those required by the pharmaceutical company sponsoring a trial, which will vary from sponsor to sponsor.

Regulatory Authorities

The FDA, a division within the Department of Health and Human Services (HHS), has the authority to enforce the laws applicable to clinical studies of investigational products. The FDA also works with its foreign regulatory counterparts to ensure that imported products comply with U.S. regulations. Sponsors must also work with foreign regulatory agencies when conducting international trials, to be sure that both U.S. and country-specific regulations are met. The sidebar on the next page lists the FDA and several (but not all) of their regulatory counterparts outside the United States.

Guidelines

Guidelines for good clinical practice are recommendations for how clinical research should be conducted. Many guidelines originated from a specific country's internal regulatory agency, while other guidelines result from work done to harmonize regulatory requirements between countries.

Regulatory Authorities

United States
Food and Drug Administration (FDA)

Canada
Health Protection Branch (HPB)

United Kingdom
Committee on Safety of Medicines (CSM)

Japan
Ministry of Health and Welfare (MHW)

European Union (EU)
Committee for Proprietary Medicinal Products (CPMP)

Germany
Bundestinstitut fur Azneimettel und Modezen Produkte (BfArM)

The European community pioneered this harmonization effort in the 1980s as European countries moved toward the development of a single market in the pharmaceutical industry. Once success was demonstrated in Europe, representatives from the regulatory and industry associations of Europe, Japan, and the United States identified the broader goal of establishing common worldwide regulations and guidelines.

At the 1990 *International Conference on Harmonization (ICH) of Technical Requirements for Registration of Pharmaceuticals for Human Use*, a committee of representatives from industry and regulatory agencies was established. This committee was charged with developing international standards that would promote greater harmonization of technical guidelines, and requirements for product registration that would prevent or reduce unnecessary duplication of testing in the development of new products without compromising safety and effectiveness. This committee's work resulted in the "ICH Guideline for Good Clinical Practice."

ICH Efficacy Guidelines

E1 Exposure

E2 Clinical safety

E3 Study reports

E4 Dose response

E5 Ethnic factors

E6 **Good clinical practice**

E7 Special populations

E8 Clinical trial design—general considerations

E9 Clinical trial design—statistical considerations

E10 Clinical trial design—choice of control group

E11 Clinical trial design—pediatric considerations

E12 Antihypertensive considerations

Categories of ICH Guidelines

ICH guidelines have been and continue to be developed in major categories including:

1 chemical and pharmaceutical quality assurance,

2 safety in pre-clinical studies,

3 efficacy of clinical studies, and

4 multidisciplinary topics such as medical terminology and electronic standards for transmission of regulatory documents.

As ICH guidelines are created and disseminated, individual countries choose whether to adopt the guidelines as established. In the United States, the FDA has adopted a number of ICH guidelines, including *E6: Good Clinical Practice*, recommending (but not requiring) investigative sites to conduct clinical research according to this guideline. E6 was adopted by the FDA and published in the May 9, 1997 Federal Register as "The ICH Guideline for Good Clinical Practice, E6."

FDA Guidances

The FDA has established documents that provide guidance about the regulations. These "Guidance Documents" are not legal requirements but serve to clarify and provide examples of ways the regulations can be met. Information Sheets have been written to clarify and/or provide additional information pertaining to the laws regulating clinical research. These Information Sheets cover wide range of topics, some of which are:

- Informed consent

- IRB operations

- Emergency use of investigational treatments

- Confidentiality

- Compensation for research-related injuries

- Frequently asked questions

- Medical devices

Local Laws

A number of cities, regions, and states in the U.S. have additional requirements for clinical research conducted within their boundaries. Local laws may cover a broad range of clinical research topics, including the age of consent, children's assent, confidentiality of patient records, institutional review boards, and vulnerable subjects.

Specific Local Laws

Currently in the state of **Massachusetts**, all investigational drugs fall into the category of controlled substances. Because of this, investigators participating in clinical trials of an investigational drug must submit a completed Massachusetts Controlled Substance Registration and a Massachusetts Registration to Conduct Research. Yearly inspections of study sites are required; an inspection is not transferable to another location even if the investigator is the same. All IRBs must be in affiliation with the state's Division of Food and Drug; it is the site investigator's responsibility to ensure this affiliation.

New York state law now requires that investigators enrolling state residents must obtain written informed consent from subjects whose blood may be screened to determine HIV status. The state of New York also has its own laboratory certification and licensure procedures that have as high or higher standards than those required by the Clinical Laboratory Improvement Amendments (CLIA) of 1988. Because of this, CLIA certification is not required for a laboratory licensed in the state of New York.

Experimental Subject's Bill of Rights

Any person who is asked to consent to participate as a human subject in medical investigation or who is asked to consent on behalf of another has the following rights:

1 To be told what the study is trying to find out.

2 To be told what will happen in the study and whether any of the procedures, drugs, or devices is different from what would be used in standard medical practice.

3 To be told about the risks, side effects, or discomforts which may be expected.

4 To be told if any benefit can be expected from participating and if so, what the benefit might be.

5 To be told of other choices available and how they may be better or worse than being in the study.

6 To be allowed to ask any questions concerning the study, both before agreeing to be involved and anytime during the course of the study.

7 To be told of any medical treatment available if complications arise.

8 To refuse to participate at all, either before or after the study has started. This decision will not affect any right to receive standard medical treatment.

9 To receive a signed and dated copy of the consent form and the Bill of Rights.

10 To be allowed time to decide to consent or not to consent to participate without any pressure being brought by the investigators or others.

The state of **California** requires that all study subjects be given a copy of the *Experimental Subject's Bill of Rights*. California law also addresses the exclusion of women and minorities in clinical research, and because of California's large non-English speaking population, places significant emphasis on translating consent forms into a subject's native language. While federal regulations require that a copy of the consent form be given to each subject, California law requires that it be a copy of the actual consent form *signed by the subject* (also recommended by ICH guidelines).

Where to Obtain Information

A number of sources provide information about the regulations and guidelines that apply to clinical research. These include the Code of Federal Regulations, the Federal Register, and FDA Guidance Documents and Information Sheets. Information can be obtained by directly contacting the FDA offices located in Rockville, Maryland, or by checking the FDA website (www.fda.gov). Local or institutional IRBs can provide information about additional requirements for local and state authorities.

The Federal Register

The Federal Register is a weekly disclosure publication that documents approved regulations. It also identifies proposed regulations, giving interested parties the opportunity to review them before they are final. Reviewers may submit comments about the content and exact wording of the regulation, the date the proposed regulation goes into effect, and the penalties for non-compliance with the regulation. Once these comments are reviewed in a government forum, the final regulation, known as a "Final Rule," is incorporated into the next issue of the Code of Federal Regulations. Revisions to Title 21 of the CFR are published annually on April 1st; Title 45 revisions are published on October 1st each year.

Useful Internet Addresses

Food and Drug Administration
http://www.fda.gov

Code of Federal Regulations
http://www.access.gpo.gov/nara/cfr/cfr-table-search.html

Federal Register
http://www.nara.gov/fedreg/

ICH Guidelines
http://www.ifpma.org/ich1.html

Internet

The Federal Register, FDA Information Sheets and Guidance Documents, the regulations, and ICH guidelines can currently be found on the Internet. The FDA website includes information on many FDA-related topics, including current product approvals, adverse reactions, FDA history, MedWatch, and recent news releases, as well as links to many other pertinent sites.

Responsibilities Identified in the Code of Federal Regulations

The regulations are a system of shared responsibilities created to conduct clinical research fairly and ethically. The FDA shares these responsibilities with the clinical investigator at the site (principal investigator), IRBs, and the study sponsor. General responsibilities for principal investigators, IRBs, and study sponsors are included in Title 21 of the Code of Federal Regulations. Federally funded studies fall under the jurisdiction of the National Institutes of Health and are also bound by the regulations in Title 45 Part 46.

The following information summarizes the responsibilities listed in the regulations; excerpts of the CFR are provided in Appendix C. It is also important to determine whether ICH guidelines must also be met (if specified by the sponsor or in the protocol). Refer to Appendix D for a listing of ICH guidelines.

Principal Investigator Responsibilities

Investigator is defined in the regulations as the "individual who actually conducts a clinical investigation (i.e., under whose immediate direction the test article is administered or dispensed to, or used involving, a subject) or, in the event of an investigation conducted by a team of individuals, is the responsible leader of that team."[1]

Responsibilities of investigators participating in investigational drug trials are listed in 21CFR § 312.60

through 312.69; those for investigators in device trials can be found in 21 CFR § 812.100 through 812.119. General responsibilities for both include conducting the study according to the protocol, obtaining IRB approval to conduct the study, obtaining informed consent from subjects before initiating study procedures, reporting adverse events, and maintaining accurate study records and drug accountability records. It is also important to refer to local rules and regulations for additional responsibilities in addition to those identified in the Code of Federal Regulations.

Investigational Drug Studies

The principal investigator is responsible for reading and understanding the protocol and the investigator's brochure. Before a clinical trial involving an investigational drug can be conducted at a site, the investigator must sign a Form FDA 1572, a contract between the FDA and the investigator (1572 is not required for device trials). When signing the required Form FDA 1572, the investigator agrees to:

1 personally conduct or supervise the study in accordance with the protocol except when necessary to protect the safety, rights, or welfare of subjects;

2 meet the requirements for obtaining informed consent;

3 report adverse experiences to the sponsor;

4 maintain adequate and accurate records and make them available for inspection;

5 ensure all associates, colleagues, and employees assisting in the conduct of the study are informed about their obligations in meeting the above commitments;

Form FDA 1572

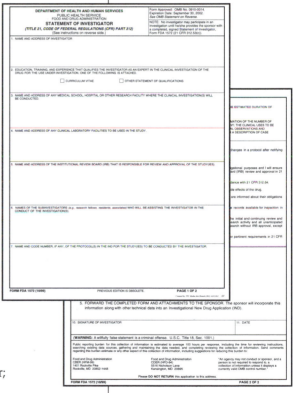

6 ensure that the IRB complies with its requirements;

7 promptly report to the IRB all changes in the research activity and all unanticipated problems related to the study; changes in the research will not be made without IRB approval except where necessary to eliminate immediate hazards to subjects;

8 comply with all other requirements regarding the obligations of clinical investigators and all other pertinent requirements in 21 CFR § 312.

General Investigator Responsibilities for Drug and Device Trials

For a full listing of specific responsibilities, refer to Title 21 of the CFR.

Maintain professional credentials
- Update CV
- Maintain expertise in clinical and research areas

Adhere to protocol
- Instruct and personally supervise staff to ensure compliance
- Ensure subjects meet eligibility criteria
- Maintain subject case records

Recruit and enroll appropriate subjects
- Ensure that selection process avoids bias
- Adhere to randomization scheme and blinding

Maintain appropriate source documentation
- Ensure that medical records reflect complete patient information
- Ensure that sponsor and regulatory authorities have access to source documents when needed

Ensure data quality
- Confirm that data are complete and accurate
- Provide timely and accurate responses to data queries

Maintain drug/device accountability
- Accurately document study drug/device received, dispensed, returned or destroyed
- Provide secure storage of study drug/device to meet specified requirements

Maintain proper study files and documentation
- Document personal involvement and tasks delegated to staff
- Document supervision/guidance to staff

Communicate with IRB
- Submit protocol, amendments, consent form, and advertising material to IRB for review and approval
- Obtain IRB approval before enrolling subjects
- Notify IRB of serious adverse events
- Provide required progress reports to IRB
- Meet IRB-required conditions of renewal
- Maintain record of all communication with IRB

Investigational Device Exemption (IDE) Studies

Responsibilities of investigators participating in IDE studies are similar to those of investigators in drug studies. In general, the investigator is responsible for ensuring that the study is conducted according to the signed agreement, the investigational plan, and applicable FDA regulations; for protecting the rights, safety, and welfare of subjects; and for the control of the device under investigation.

Unlike investigational drug trials, however, investigators participating in IDE studies are not required to sign a Form FDA 1572 or other such form listing these responsibilities. Much of the same information recorded on a Form FDA 1572 (name and address of investigator and institution) must be provided to the FDA as part of the IDE application; however, the sponsor may collect this information in their own format.

Institutional Review Board (IRB) Responsibilities

An institutional review board refers to any board, committee, or other group that has the responsibility to review, approve the initiation of, and to conduct periodic review of biomedical research involving human subjects.[2] The primary purpose of the IRB review process is to assure that the rights and welfare of human subjects are protected.

An IRB may invite individuals with competence in specific areas to participate in

---

Some of the IRB Responsibilities for Studies of Drugs, Biologics, and Devices:

1 Reviewing, approving/disapproving, or requiring modification of all research activities covered by the regulations;

2 Requiring documentation of informed consent in accordance with the regulations, except in the cases when written consent can be waived for some or all subjects because research activities present no more than minimal risk of harm and involve no procedures for which written consent is required outside the research context;

3 Providing investigators and institutions with written documentation of approval, disapproval, and/or required modifications of all research activities;

4 Reviewing the research at least once a year in accordance with the regulations;

5 Ensuring that IRB committee membership consists of at least five members:

- who have no conflicting interest in any project reviewed by the IRB;

- of both sexes, when possible, and sufficiently qualified with different backgrounds, expertise, experience, and diversity;

- at least one of whom is not employed by or otherwise affiliated with the institution; this member may not be part of the immediate family of someone employed by or affiliated with the institution;

- one whose primary concern or work is in a scientific area; and

- one whose primary concern or work is non-scientific.

A full list of responsibilities can be found in Title 21 Part 56.

the review of complex issues beyond the expertise of IRB members, but these individuals cannot vote with the IRB. An IRB must conduct continuing review of previously approved protocols at intervals appropriate to the degree of risk involved in the study, but no less than once a year. An IRB can perform expedited review of a study if there is no more than minimal risk or if there are minor changes to a study approved in the previous 12 months.

Additional IRB Responsibilities for IDE Trials

IRBs reviewing IDE trials must comply with the requirements of 21 CFR § 56 and have the additional responsibilities that are found in the device regulations in 21 CFR § 812.60–66. The IRB also assesses whether a device meets the definitions of non-significant versus significant risk. This distinction regarding risk is important, since NSR devices are governed by different regulations and are subject to abbreviated requirements [21 CFR § 812.2(b)]; sponsors are not required to submit an IDE application or notify the FDA before starting an NSR device study. When the sponsor submits an NSR device study to an IRB for review, the IRB must first determine if it is in agreement with the risk assessment, and subsequently approve or disapprove of the study. If the IRB disagrees with the sponsor's NSR assessment, the sponsor must then submit an IDE application to the FDA before conducting the study. See Chapter 2 for additional information about significant risk and non-significant risk devices.

Sponsor Responsibilities

The regulations define a sponsor as the "person or other entity that initiates a clinical investigation, but that does not actually conduct the investigation, i.e., the test article is administered or dispensed to, or used involving, a subject under the immediate direction of another individual."[3]

Sponsors may transfer any or all responsibilities to a contract or academic organization; however, any such transfer must be described in writing. The organization assuming the responsibilities transferred from the sponsor must comply with all applicable regulations and is subject to the same regulatory action as a sponsor for failure to comply.

As part of the sponsor's responsibilities for ongoing review, a sponsor who discovers that an investigator is not complying with the Form FDA 1572, the study protocol, or the regulations shall either secure compliance from the investigator or end the investigator's participation in the study. Ending the investigator's participation includes discontinuing shipment of study materials to the investigator, requiring the investigator to return remaining products, and notifying the FDA.

Sponsor Responsibilities in IDE Studies

Sponsor responsibilities for device trials are listed in 21 CFR Subpart C, 812.40 through 812.47, and are similar to those for investigational drug studies. Instead of an IND, the sponsor submits an IDE application, and is responsible for selecting qualified investigators and keeping them informed about the study, ensuring proper monitoring of the study, ensuring that IRB review and approval is obtained, and ensuring that all reviewing IRBs and the FDA are promptly informed of significant new information about the study. Financial disclosure information about participating investigators and the reporting of unanticipated adverse device effects must also be submitted to the FDA.

Financial Disclosure Regulations

Financial disclosure regulations effective as of February 2, 1999, require the party who submits the marketing

Among the sponsor responsibilities for studies involving investigational drugs identified in 21 CFR § 312.50 through 312.59 are:

1   selecting qualified investigators (qualified by training and experience as appropriate experts to investigate the investigational product);

2   providing investigators with information to conduct the study properly;

3   ensuring proper monitoring (study conducted per protocol and with applicable ethical and regulatory considerations);

4   ensuring the study is conducted according to the general plan and protocols contained in the Investigational New Drug (IND) application;

5   maintaining an effective IND with respect to the study and protocol;

6   ensuring that the FDA and all participating investigators are promptly informed of significant new adverse effects/risks with respect to the drug;

7   submitting financial disclosure information via Form FDA 3453 and/or 3455 regarding the financial interests of each participating investigator.

- Stock in the sponsoring company

- Proprietary interest (e.g., patent, trademark, copyright, licensing agreement)

- Payment arrangements that benefit the investigator if a certain study outcome occurs

- Honoraria

- Gifts of equipment

- Retainers for ongoing consultation

application (New Drug Application or Investigational Device Exemption application) to the FDA, to certify the absence of financial interest of any clinical investigator conducting the studies or disclose those interests if they exist. This rule is intended to identify potential bias of investigators due to financial interest.

Clinical investigators as defined by this rule include the listed or identified investigators or sub-investigators who are directly involved in the treatment or evaluation of research subjects. Financial disclosure is also required for the spouses and dependent children of the identified investigators.[4] When a Form FDA 1572 is completed for a trial conducted under an IND, financial disclosure should be provided for the principal investigator identified in section #1 on Form FDA 1572, all persons listed as subinvestigators in section #6, as well as the spouses and dependent children of all investigators in both sections. For device trials where there is no Form FDA 1572, the investigator(s) designated in the IDE application should provide financial disclosure information. Investigators are required to disclose compensation affected by the outcome of the study, significant payments (currently > \$25,000) from the sponsor excluding the cost of conducting the study, proprietary interest in the tested product, and significant equity interest (currently > \$50,000) in the sponsor.

Generally, the financial disclosure information should be collected before shipment of the test article to the investigators. If the party submitting the marketing application does not include either certification and/or disclosure of investigators, or does not certify that it was not possible to obtain this information, the FDA may refuse the marketing application.

Federally Funded Clinical Trials

When clinical studies are conducted by the Department of Health and Human Services (HHS) or funded in whole or part by the HHS, these studies fall under the regulations found in Part 46 of Title 45 of the Code of Federal Regulations. As the federal government's primary agency for advancing knowledge in the biomedical and behavioral sciences to understand and treat human disease, the National Institutes of Health (NIH) conducts clinical trials under this title of the CFR. When the NIH collaborates with and/or provides funding for clinical trials at institutions outside the NIH, those institutions are also bound to follow the regulations put forth in Title 45, Part 46.

When studies involving products regulated by the FDA are funded, supported, or conducted by the FDA and/or the NIH, both the HHS regulations (Title 45) and FDA regulations (Title 21) apply.

	FDA – Title 21	HHS – Title 45
IRB Assurance Mechanism	56.115 — FDA does not have an assurance mechanism nor files of IRB membership.	46.115 — HHS has IRB assurance mechanism and requires notification of IRB membership changes.
Informed Consent	50.23 — FDA provides for an exception from the informed consent requirements in emergency situations.	HHS does not provide for this exception.
Informed Consent Elements	FDA has no provision to alter or waive elements of informed consent because the types of studies that would qualify for such waivers are either not regulated by the FDA or are covered by the emergency treatment provisions (50.23).	46.11(c) and (d) — HHS provides for waiving or altering elements of informed consent under certain conditions.
Consent Forms	50.27 — FDA explicitly requires that consent forms be dated as well as signed by the subject or subject's legally authorized representative.	HHS regulations do not explicitly require consent forms to be dated.

Vulnerable Subjects

When **prisoners** are subjects of a federally funded study, Title 45 requires that at least one member of the reviewing IRB shall be a prisoner, or a prisoner representative with appropriate background and experience to serve in that capacity [45 CFR § 46.304(b)].

No **pregnant woman** may be involved as a subject unless 1) the purpose of the activity is to meet the health needs of the mother and the fetus will be placed at risk only to the minimum extent necessary to meet such needs, or 2) the risk to the fetus is minimal [45 CFR § 46.207(a)]. HHS is currently reviewing its regulations regarding pregnant women and fetuses to make these rules more inclusive. Consult 45 CFR § 46 Subpart B for the latest revisions.

When **children** are subjects in a clinical trial, there must be provisions made to solicit the assent of the children, when in the judgment of the IRB, the children are capable of providing assent [45 CFR § 46.408 and 21 CFR § 50.55]. (See Chapter 4 for information on assent of children.)

Differences Between CFR Title 21 and Title 45

Title 21 and Title 45 of the CFR both embody the ethical principles of the Belmont Report, serving as a framework to ensure that serious efforts have been made to protect the rights and welfare of human subjects. There are, however, differences in the regulations found in Titles 21 and 45. Some of these differences are listed in the table on page 49.

There are also special considerations provided in Title 45 for groups of subjects who are considered to be more vulnerable. These include pregnant women, fetuses, and prisoners. The regulations safeguarding these groups can be found in 45 CFR § 46 Subparts B and C and pertain to subjects in federally funded clinical trials. Under an interim rule effective April 30, 2001, in 21 CFR § 50 Subpart D, there are now safeguards for children as a vulnerable group that mirror those previously found only in Title 45.

In June 2000, the NIH released notices containing changes and clarifications of policies regarding training of investigators involved in clinical research and data and safety monitoring in clinical trials. These notices apply to studies conducted under Title 45.

- **Training:** All new and non-competing grant applications submitted after October 1, 2000, must indicate that all key personnel involved in the research have received training in the protection of human subjects.

- **Data and Safety Monitoring:** Requires investigators to submit data and safety monitoring plans for Phase I and Phase II trials, in addition to Phase III trials, which were required prior to this.

While sponsors of studies conducted under Title 21 may require investigator education or provide for data and safety monitoring in Phase I and II trials, it is currently not a regulatory requirement of non-federally funded trials under the jurisdiction of the FDA.

Assurance of Compliance

When an institution applies for federal funding for a research project, such as through the NIH, it must complete a written agreement stating that it will comply with the regulatory requirements in *Title 45, Part 46, Public Welfare*. The written document is referred to as an "assurance of compliance" (commonly referred to as an "assurance") and is an agreement between the institution and the Office for Human Research Protections (OHRP). The assurance formally acknowledges the institution's commitment to conduct research under the basic ethical principles and to comply with the regulations. The OHRP, formerly called the Office for Protection from Research Risks (OPRR), is responsible for interpreting and overseeing the implementation of the regulations regarding the protection of human subjects (45 CFR § 46) and for providing guidance on ethical issues. This role extends to all institutions where federal funds are used to conduct or support clinical research.

A Multiple-Project Assurance (MPA) is an assurance that extends to the conduct of more than one clinical research study at an institution. Multiple project assurances are issued by the OHRP for multi-year periods of time. A Single-Project Assurance (SPA) is submitted when an institution does not have or need an assurance for multiple projects. The SPA is applicable only to the single designated project.

References

1 21 CFR § 56.102(h) and 21 CFR § 812.3 (i)

2 21 CFR § 56.102(g)

3 21 CFR § 56.102(j)

4 21 CFR § 54.2(d)

"For knowledge, too, is itself power."

—*Francis Bacon, Mediatationes Sacrae*

Informed Consent and the Regulations

For specific instructions and responsibilities regarding informed consent, refer to the Code of Federal Regulations, FDA Information Sheets and Guidance Documents, and ICH guidelines.

What Is Informed Consent?

Informed consent is the process of providing information to a potential subject in such a manner that the subject is given adequate time and information to make an informed decision about study participation.

Informed consent is based on three elements:

1 information about the proposed research study;

2 comprehension of that information; and

3 voluntary participation.

Regulations regarding informed consent can be found in Title 21, Part 50, Subpart B—Informed Consent of Human Subjects. When obtaining assent from children as subjects in clinical trials, refer to Title 45 Part 46, Subpart D—Additional Protections for Children Involved as Subjects in Research and to the interim rule in Title 21, Part 50, Subpart D—Additional Safeguards for Children in Clinical Investigations. Additional safeguards for the protection of pregnant women and fetuses, and for prisoners participating in federally funded research that affect informed consent can be found in 45 CFR § 46, Subparts B and C.

These regulations are intended to safeguard the rights and welfare of subjects participating in clinical research and are applicable to studies of drugs, biologics, and devices. Informed consent must also be obtained when studies do not involve the use of a medical product, but are conducted to solicit information from subjects, such as the administration of questionnaires, the retrospective review and recording of medical record data, or comparison of activities (e.g., exercise versus meditation).

Informed Consent:
A subject's voluntary agreement to participate in a clinical research study after receiving and comprehending information about the study, including the risks and benefits of participation, and alternative therapy if unwilling to participate.

As is evident in the regulated responsibilities for investigators, IRBs, and sponsors (Chapter 3), all three groups are responsible for ensuring the ethical conduct of a study, which includes informed consent. A number of codes of medical ethics stress the personal responsibility of physician-investigators to provide their patients with adequate and appropriate information. The Declaration of Helsinki and the Belmont Report (see Appendix A) both identify ethical conduct for experiments in humans. Ethical conduct issues revolve around the safety of the participating individual rather than the community at large. Although the community may benefit from an individual's participation in clinical research, an individual should not be subjected to unreasonable harm or risk for the sake of the community.

In addition to these ethical codes of conduct, laws contained in the Code of Federal Regulations regulate how consent is obtained from study participants. Two primary historical events that have shaped the current process are the medical experiments performed on prisoners-of-war during World War II and the Tuskegee Syphilis Study conducted under the U.S. Public Health Service.

Regulations have since been implemented to ensure that all future study participants are given sufficient information about the study, study procedures, and alternative treatment, and given a choice of whether or not to participate. The regulations require that information be presented in a manner and at a level that subjects can comprehend.

The informed consent process usually begins by providing a potential subject with both verbal and written information about the study. Adequate time for questions and answers should be allowed, giving the potential subject time to review the written consent form that provides study-specific information and to make a decision about study participation. While the written consent form

During the trial of 23 Nazi physicians held at Nuremberg in 1946, fundamental ethical standards for the conduct of human research were documented in the Nuremberg Code, setting forth ten conditions that must be met to justify research involving human subjects. One of the most important conditions was the need for voluntary informed consent from subjects.

In the 1970s it was discovered that since the 1930s, approximately 400 African-American men with syphilis had been involved, without their knowledge, in a study on the natural course of the disease. In this study performed in Tuskegee, Alabama, these men were denied treatment with penicillin to allow researchers to follow the progression of untreated syphilis.

provides documentation of the process, it does not replace the discussion that should occur between a potential study participant and the individual obtaining consent. Exceptions to this process include life-threatening situations when there is not adequate time to review the details of the study and there is no alternative life-saving treatment.

It is important for both the investigator and the study participant to understand that informed consent is an ongoing process that does not end with a signature on a written consent form, but continues through completion of study procedures and follow-up. Study participants should be informed about the occurrence of new developments that may affect their decision to continue participation in the study.

A summary of the requirements regarding informed consent and exceptions to the general requirements for informed consent can be found on the following page with the regulations provided in Appendix C.

Informed Consent Process

A Consent Form is provided by the sponsor with the study protocol or created by the site investigator.

The Consent Form is personalized by each site, adding local contact names and numbers.

The Consent Form is approved for use by the Institutional Review Board.

Investigator or designated study personnel inform the patient about the study purpose, risks, and potential benefits.

The patient is allowed time to read the Consent Form, ask questions, and consider participation.

The patient or legal representative signs and dates* the Consent Form. The sponsor and/or IRB may require additional signatures.

The patient is given a copy of the Consent Form and study treatment and procedures can be started.

* Date not required for Title 45 trials

> Informed Consent is an *ongoing process*. The patient should be provided with information throughout the study that might influence the patient's decision to continue participation.

1. Source documents must reflect that consent was obtained before the start of study treatment and procedures.

2. A copy of the signed consent form must be kept at the site.

3. All versions of approved consent forms must be kept in the site file; only the current IRB-approved version may be used to consent new patients.

General Requirements for Informed Consent

(21 CFR § 50.20)

The following summary lists the general requirements of informed consent from Title 21 of the Code of Federal Regulations.

1 No investigator may involve a human subject in a clinical trial unless legally effective informed consent has first been obtained (except as provided in 21 CFR § 50.23; see below).

2 The subject or the subject's legal representative must be provided sufficient opportunity to consider whether or not to participate, with minimal coercion or undue influence.

3 Information presented to the subject must be in language understandable to the subject or representative (as determined by the IRB and local community needs).

4 No consent form may include exculpatory language through which the subject or legal representative waives or appears to waive any legal rights or releases or appears to release the investigator, sponsor, the institution, or its agent from liability for negligence.[1]

Exceptions from the General Requirements

(21 CFR § 50.23)

There are some situations in which the general requirements for informed consent do not apply and a waiver of the requirements may be requested. An example of a situation in which general requirements might be waived is the unconscious patient admitted to an emergency department whose only chance of survival is to receive an investigational treatment.

All four of the following must be true to request consideration for waiving the requirements:

1 the subject is confronted by a life-threatening situation and administration of the study treatment may save the subject's life; and

2 informed consent cannot be obtained because of the subject's inability to communicate or give consent; and

3 there is not sufficient time to obtain consent from the subject's legal representative; and

4 there is no alternative treatment available that is likely to provide an equal or greater chance of saving the subject's life.

To satisfy the regulations regarding waiving the general requirements, these four conditions must be certified in writing by the investigator and a physician not participating in the study. Written certification must be submitted to the IRB within five working days after investigational treatment was administered.

The **MAGIC** (**MAG**nesium **I**n **C**ardiac arrest) trial was conducted at Duke University Hospital. Eligible patients were at least 18 years of age and had been treated by the hospital code team for cardiac arrest, defined as the cessation of cardiac mechanical activity confirmed by the absence of consciousness, spontaneous respiration, blood pressure, and pulse. The IRB waived the requirement for informed consent for the MAGIC trial in accordance with the regulatory guidelines.

The decision to waive requirements was based on the following: unconscious patients are not able to give consent, the delay required to obtain consent from family members would diminish the treatment's potential efficacy, eligible patients could not be reliably identified before arrest, and the research project was deemed to be in the patients' best interest and reasonably comparable to available interventions. These patients were in a life-threatening situation, available treatments were unsatisfactory, and clinical investigation was required to determine the efficacy of the treatment.

Elements of Informed Consent

(21 CFR § 50.25)

The regulations identify eight "basic" elements that must be included in every consent form. In addition to these basic elements, the regulations identify six "additional" elements that must be included when appropriate. These elements are summarized on the next page and can be found in Title 21 of the Code of Federal Regulations, Part 50.25 (see Appendix C). These elements are based on the following ethical considerations:

- participation in a clinical trial should be voluntary and potential enrollees should not be pressured to participate;

- subjects should be allowed to withdraw from the study without penalty;

- subjects should be capable of making a rational decision to participate;

- subjects should be reasonably informed although they need not understand all the scientific principles pertaining to the study;

- certain categories of subjects are considered vulnerable and require special consideration as to whether they are capable of giving rational informed consent to participate. Subjects considered to be vulnerable include prisoners, infants and children, pregnant women, and mentally disabled persons.[2]

Synopsis of Elements

Basic Elements

1. Statement that study involves research and explanation of procedures

2. Description of reasonably foreseeable risks

3. Description of benefits

4. Alternative procedures or courses of treatment

5. Description of confidentiality of records

6. Explanation of compensation and medical treatment for injury occurring during study

7. Contact persons for study questions and research-related injury

8. Statement that participation is voluntary and that there is no penalty or loss of benefits for refusal to participate

Additional Elements

1. Statement of unforeseeable risks to subject, embryo, or fetus

2. Circumstances of subject participation termination by investigator

3. Additional costs to subject

4. Consequences of and procedures for withdrawal (e.g., tapering drug)

5. Statement about informing subject of significant new findings that might affect subject's willingness to participate

6. Approximate number of subjects

Whereas the CFR identifies these eight basic elements and six additional elements of informed consent, the ICH guidelines identify 20 essential elements of informed consent (see Appendix D).

Documentation of Informed Consent

(21 CFR § 50.27)

Informed consent must be documented in a written consent form approved by the IRB except as provided in 21 CFR § 56.109(c).[3] The consent form must be signed by the subject or the subject's legal representative (as defined by each state) and a copy given to the person signing the form.

Except as provided in 21 CFR § 56.109(c), the consent form may be either:

1 a written consent form that includes the basic and applicable additional elements of informed consent; the form may be read by the subject or representative, or read to the subject or representative if appropriate;

2 a "short form" written consent document that states that the elements of informed consent have been presented orally to the subject or representative. When this method is used, there must be a witness to the oral presentation and a written summary of what is said.

Written Consent Forms

The written consent form must contain the eight *Basic Elements of Informed Consent* and any of the *Additional Elements of Informed Consent* that are applicable (see Appendix B for a sample consent form). When adhering to ICH guidelines for informed consent, the consent form must contain all 20 elements identified in the ICH guidelines. When a subject agrees to participate, the subject or subject's legal representative must sign the consent form indicating willingness to participate in the study. The CFR regulations require that a copy of the consent form be given to the subject. While the federal regulations do not require this to be a copy of the consent form with the patient's signature, the ICH guidelines, as well as some states and local IRBs, do have this requirement.

If a subject is not able to read, the consent form may be read aloud verbatim to patients. When a subject does not speak English, the consent form should be translated into the language understood by the subject.

21 CFR § 56.109(c):
An IRB shall require documentation of informed consent in accordance with 50.27, except that the IRB may, for some or all subjects, waive the requirement that the subject or the subject's legally authorized representative sign a written consent form if it finds that the research presents no more than minimal risk of harm to subjects and involves no procedures for which written consent is normally required outside the research context. In cases where the documentation requirement is waived, the IRB may require the investigator to provide subjects with a written statement regarding the research.

4. Informed Consent and The Regulations

61

Short Form

The "short form" is an alternative to the traditional written consent form containing details of the study information. The "short" consent form simply states that the elements of informed consent have been orally presented to the patient or the patient's legal representative. When a short form is used, there must be an impartial witness to the oral presentation to verify that all of the required elements of informed consent were presented. A short form must be approved by the Institutional Review Board (IRB) before use and signed by both the patient and the witness.

A written summary of the information to be presented must also be approved by the IRB if a short form is being used. When discussing study participation with a potential subject, information should not be given extemporaneously or

Sample Short Form

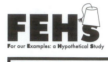

Consent to Participate in a Research Study: Short Form

Study Name:	FEHS (For our Examples: a Hypothetical Study)
Protocol Number	XYZ 39-90213
Date:	September 11, 1999
Sponsor:	Pharmaceutical Company, USA
Principal Investigator:	_____
Institution:	_____

I give my consent to participate in this research study that is being done to compare an investigational clot-dissolving medicine to one already on the market. All the items on the Written Summary have been explained to me in the presence of a witness. These include the background and purpose of the study, the procedures required for the study, possible risks and benefits, alternative treatment if I do not participate, confidentiality of my records, compensation, and the names of those I should contact if I have any questions. It has been explained that it is up to me to decide if I want to participate in the study. If I do participate, pertinent new information will be explained to me while I am in the study. I have had the chance to ask questions and they have all been answered so that I understand. I have been told that a copy of this consent form and a copy of the written summary will be given to me.

```
_____     _____     _/_/_
Name of Study Participant   Signature of Study Participant   Date
```

I have witnessed the summary information being verbally presented to the subject. I confirm that all of the information in the written summary has been completely and accurately explained. The subject was given time to ask questions and the questions were answered so that the subject could understand. The subject voluntarily agreed to participate in this study and signed/marked this consent form.

```
_____     _____     _/_/_
Name of Witness           Signature of Witness          Date
```

	Short Form	Written Summary
IRB	Must approve	Must approve
Subject	Must sign, gets a copy	Gets a copy
Person obtaining consent		Must sign
Witness	Must sign	Must sign

from memory. The individual presenting the information to the patient or representative should use the written summary while orally presenting the study to ensure that the same information is presented to all potential subjects, and that all points are reviewed. Both the person presenting the information and the witness to the presentation must sign the written summary. The subject or representative must be given a copy of both the short form and the written summary.

Short forms are typically used in trials where study patients are acutely ill. Since it is unlikely that an acutely ill patient who is experiencing severe pain or other significant symptoms could carefully read and consider all the aspects of study participation, the short form presentation is an appropriate alternative to the written form. In situations such as these, when time-to-treatment is especially critical, the informed consent process can be fulfilled by reviewing the pertinent aspects of the study identified on the written summary associated with the study short form.

Sample Written Summary of a Research Study

FEHs
For our Examples: a Hypothetical Study

Written Summary

1 Since your doctor has determined that you are having a heart attack, you are being asked to participate in this research study.

2 Your participation is completely voluntary and if you decide to participate, you may withdraw your consent at any time without jeopardy to your medical care.

BACKGROUND AND PURPOSE OF STUDY

3 This study is being done to see if an investigational clot-dissolving medicine is as good as or better than a similar medicine already on the market, when given to people having a heart attack.

4 By quickly dissolving the blood clot in the arteries to the heart, the blood flow can resume and may reduce the amount of heart damage.

5 Approximately 5000 people in the United States will be enrolled in this study.

PROCEDURES

6 You will be given a dose of either the investigational clot-dissolving medicine or the medicine already in use for people with heart attacks. You have a 50% chance of getting the investigational medicine.

7 The medicine is prepared so that neither you nor your doctors know which medicine you are given.

8 The medicine will be given through your veins over one hour.

9 You will have your blood drawn before the medicine is given and again each morning that you are in the hospital. About 2 tablespoons of blood will be drawn each time.

POSSIBLE RISKS

10 All medicines that dissolve blood clots can cause internal bleeding. This could include bleeding into your brain, causing a stroke, which occurs in less than 1% of people who get clot-dissolving medicine.

11 If bleeding is severe, you may need a blood transfusion.

12 There could be side effects that we currently don't know about.

POSSIBLE BENEFITS

13 If you get the investigational medicine, it could prove to be better at dissolving the blood clot and getting the blood flowing back to your heart.

14 The marketed medicine dissolves blood clots in about 70% of people who receive it.

ALTERNATIVE TREATMENT

15 If you are not in the study, you will probably be given the marketed medicine for your heart attack.

CONFIDENTIALITY

16 Information about you and how you responded to the treatment will be recorded on forms but your name and other information identifying you will not be written on the forms.

17 The FDA and other personnel from the company who makes the investigational medicine may review your medical records to confirm the information written on the forms.

COMPENSATION

18 You will not receive money or any other kind of compensation or reward for being in the study.

19 You will receive the clot-dissolving medicine and the blood tests required for this study for free; you or your insurance will be billed for the rest of your hospital charges.

20 If you have an injury because of being in this study, you will receive free medical care for the injury.

CONTACTS

21 If you have any questions about the study, you should call Dr. Knowledge at (888) 111-2222. If you have any questions about your rights as a participant in a research study, you should call Ms. Answers, the chairperson of the hospital committee that reviews research studies, at (888) 333-4444.

OTHER

22 If your doctor or the company that makes the investigational medicine thinks your health or safety could be harmed if you continue in the study, your participation will be stopped.

23 While you are in the study, you will be told about any new information that might make you change your mind about participating in the study.

SIGNATURES

I confirm that the information in this written summary has been verbally presented to the subject and that consent to participate has been freely given by the subject.

Name of Witness

Signature of Witness _____ __/__/__ Date

Name of Person Obtaining Consent

Signature of Person Obtaining Consent _____ __/__/__ Date

Consent from Vulnerable Subjects

Certain groups of subjects are considered to be more vulnerable, requiring special protection to maintain their rights and safety. These groups include children, pregnant women, fetuses, and prisoners. The Belmont Report (Appendix A) contains a comprehensive discussion of the issues related to the vulnerability of these groups of individuals.

Regulations for Consent

Specific regulations regarding informed consent for vulnerable groups of subjects participating in clinical trials can be found in Titles 21 and 45 of the Code of Federal Regulations as listed below.

Title 21, Part 50, Subpart D—Additional Safeguards for Children in Clinical Investigations (interim rule effective April 30, 2001)

Title 45, Part 46, Subpart B—Additional Protections Pertaining to Research, Development, and Related Activities Involving Fetuses, Pregnant Women, and Human In Vitro Fertilization

Title 45, Part 46, Subpart C—Additional Protections Pertaining to Biomedical and Behavioral Research Involving Prisoners as Subjects

Title 45, Part 46, Subpart D—Additional Protections for Children Involved as Subjects in Research

Assent from Children

When children are the subjects in a clinical trial, consent or "permission" for the child to participate is required from the parent or legal guardian. Depending on applicable state and local laws, parents, legal guardians, and/or others may have the ability to give permission to enroll children in a clinical study. IRBs generally require investigators to obtain the *permission* of one or both parents or guardian and the *assent* of children who possess the intellectual and emotional ability to understand the concepts involved. Older children may be familiar with signing documents through previous experience with testing, applying for a driver's license, or obtaining a passport, while younger children may never have had the experience of signing a document. Therefore, some IRBs require two consent forms: one that fully explains the study procedures for the parents and older children, and a second one that is shorter and simpler for younger children.

It is the responsibility of the IRB reviewing the protocol to determine if assent is required. The IRB will inform the investigator of additional requirements unique to children participating in research, including whether a separate consent form outlining the study in simplified language is needed.

Assent means that the child agrees to participate even though he or she may not understand all the specific information concerning the study.

References

1 21 CFR § 50.23(a)

2 Applied Clinical Trials, December 1996, Clinical Trials: An Overview

3 21 CFR § 56.109(c)

"Sweet are the uses of adversity,
Which like the toad, ugly and venomous,
Wears yet a precious jewel in his head;
And this our life, exempt from public haunt,
Finds tongues in trees, books in the running brooks,
Sermons in stones, and good in every thing."

—*William Shakespeare*, As You Like It, *Act II Scene 1*

Adverse Events

Why Collect Adverse Event Data?

One of the most important responsibilities of the site investigator is the accurate, timely, and complete reporting of adverse events. Adverse events are collected in clinical drug trials to:

1 Determine the safety profile of a drug

2 Evaluate the benefits and risks of a drug

3 Provide information for the package insert if a drug is marketed

Safety Profile

The safety profile of a drug is carefully monitored in clinical trials to determine if there are significant concerns that would prevent it from being used in the target patient population. The investigator's brochure contains all adverse events reported in trials of the drug to date, and describes the number of times specific events were reported. Sometimes drugs are found to be effective but have such serious untoward effects that further studies of the drug are discontinued.

Benefits and Risks Evaluation

The FDA recognizes the need for a medical risk-benefit judgment as part of the process of approving a drug for marketing. In this evaluation, the FDA considers whether the benefits of the drug outweigh its known and potential risks as well as the need to answer remaining questions about the drug's effectiveness.[1] Included in the FDA assessment of the risk-to-benefit ratio is a careful evaluation of all adverse events reported during clinical trials.

Package Insert

Sponsors use adverse event information to prepare the package insert for the drug. Package inserts, based on scientific facts gleaned from clinical trials, are written to help health care providers prescribe the drug for appropriate patients and inform them of potential side effects. The package insert also serves as a source document by which the FDA can evaluate additional adverse events reported after marketing.

Defining Adverse Events

An adverse event is generally defined as any unfavorable change in a patient that may occur during or after administration of a drug or device. This change does not have to be caused by the treatment to be called an adverse event.

Adverse events can be:

- Physical signs or symptoms

- Abnormal laboratory values

- Changes in vital signs, physical examination, or on an electrocardiogram

- An increase in the frequency or intensity (worsening) of a condition or illness that was present before study enrollment

- Complications from a surgery or procedure

Benefit versus Risk:

"Take AZT, for example," says Robert Temple, MD, director of the Office of Drug Evaluation I in CDER. (AZT is marketed as Retrovir and is used to treat AIDS.) "It has significant toxicity. If you weren't quite sure it had a benefit, it would be hard to describe it as 'safe.' But we know from well-controlled studies, that it has a benefit. In the first large clinical study with the drug, there were 19 deaths in patients taking a placebo, but only one death among those on AZT."

5. Adverse Events

Adverse events are not:

- Procedures or surgeries (the medical condition that caused the need for the procedure or surgery is the adverse event)

- Pre-existing events or illnesses that do not worsen during the study period

Several subsets of adverse events may be differentiated in clinical trials. These include expected versus unexpected adverse events and serious versus non-serious adverse events.

Expected versus Unexpected Adverse Events

An expected adverse event is one that is *expected for the drug* based on previous clinical experience and has been previously reported in the investigator's brochure, or on the package insert.

An unexpected adverse event is one that is *unexpected for the drug* and has not been reported in the investigator's brochure or package insert, or is an event that is being reported in greater severity or frequency than the same event previously reported.

Serious versus Non-Serious Adverse Events

A Serious Adverse Event (SAE) is defined as any experience occurring at any dose (regardless of relationship to study agent) that meets one of the following conditions:

- Results in death

- Is life-threatening

- Results in persistent or significant disability/incapacity

- Requires or prolongs inpatient hospitalization

- Is a congenital anomaly/birth defect

An important medical event that may not lead to death, be life-threatening, or require hospitalization may be also be considered a serious adverse event. This would pertain to events that, when based upon appropriate medical judgment, may jeopardize the patient or subject and may require medical or surgical intervention to prevent one of the outcomes listed above.[2]

Events that are not serious adverse events by the above definition are usually considered to be non-serious events.

Investigator Responsibilities

The investigator is responsible for collecting and reporting (to the sponsor or designee) all pertinent information about adverse events as required in the protocol.

Collecting Adverse Event Data

Adverse events may be observed by the investigator and other personnel responsible for the care of the patient, reported spontaneously by the patient, or reported in reply to open-ended questions. Observations of potential adverse events should be made objectively and thoroughly. To avoid bias, questions posed to the patient should occur in a systematic but non-specific way, such as, "Have you had any health problems or have there been any changes in the way you feel since you started the study medication?" Asking specific questions such as "Have you had any headaches?" is too specific and may be suggestive to the patient.

Reporting Adverse Event Data

Clinical trials may require a different mindset from clinical practice in reference to reporting adverse events. An event that does not require clinical treatment or is not regarded as significant by the investigator must still be reported in the trial if it meets the definitions provided. In many trials, investigators are required to report all events to the sponsor, even when in the investigator's opinion the event is not related to the investigational agent. Complete reporting is necessary because the relationship of an event to an investigational agent is not always apparent at one site, and what appears to be an isolated, unrelated event may actually be part of a larger pattern occurring in many patients at multiple sites.

There are different mechanisms for the investigator to report adverse events to the sponsor, depending on the type of adverse event, the seriousness of the event, and the process outlined for the specific study. Some events may be reported to the sponsor only by recording on the patient data forms, while other events will require expedited reporting to the sponsor via fax forms or by telephone. Adverse events that are both serious and unexpected usually need to be reported to both the sponsor and the IRB.

The protocol should identify events that need to be recorded in the patient case report forms. These forms generally collect the following types of data:

- *Event:* The adverse event should be reported in medical terminology. Depending on the sponsor and the trial, you may be asked to report the event as a diagnosis (asthma) or you may be required to report a sign or symptom (bronchospasm or wheezing).

- *Relationship to study drug (causality):* The investigator will be asked to evaluate whether the adverse event was related to, or caused by, the study drug. Typically, the investigator is asked to indicate this relationship as (1) a reasonable possibility or (2) not a reasonable possibility.

  Some sponsors may ask the investigator to further categorize this as (1) unrelated, (2) remotely related, (3) possibly related (uncertain as to relationship), (4) probably (likely) related, or (5) definitely related. The investigator may also be requested to provide a rationale to support his/her opinion.

- *Severity/intensity:* "Mild" indicates the patient was aware of the event but that it was easily tolerated. "Moderate" signifies discomfort sufficient to interfere with normal activities, while "severe" indicates the patient was incapacitated with an inability to perform normal activities.

- *Seriousness:* If the event meets one or more of the criteria in the definition of a serious adverse event, the event should be classified as serious.

The distinction between the *severity* of an event versus the *seriousness* of an event is an important distinction. While severity is based on the intensity of the event, seriousness is based upon the event outcome as it poses a threat to the patient's life or functioning. An event can be severe in intensity but not be classified a serious adverse event: For example, vomiting that persists for several hours may be considered to be of severe intensity but not a serious adverse event. While an event of mild or moderate intensity, such as a stroke resulting in a limited degree of disability, may be considered a mild stroke, it should be classified as a serious adverse event since it meets one or more of the criteria (i.e., significant disability and requires or prolongs hospitalization).

Sample Adverse Event Page

In addition to the above items, the investigator may be required to record pertinent data about the onset and resolution of the event, treatment provided in response to the event, and action taken with regard to study treatment for the patient with the event.

Expedited Reporting of Adverse Events

The protocol should identify specific adverse events that the investigator is required to report to the sponsor in an expedited manner. These events, determined through discussions between the sponsor and the FDA during the Investigational New Drug application process, often include serious adverse events that are also unexpected and related to the study treatment. The sponsor or designated group responsible for drug safety in the trial will outline a process for the expedited reporting of events. Events requiring expedited reporting are typically reported on a separate Serious Adverse Event (SAE) report form (or some other similar name), on which the investigator provides very specific information about the event. This form often includes a narrative description of the event, as well as relevant medical history, laboratory results, diagnostic tests, concomitant medications, treatment, and the outcome of the event.

The SAE report form used to report events that require expedited reporting is typically faxed to the drug safety group, usually within 24 hours of the investigator learning of the event. A phone call may also be required to report certain events, such as those leading to death.

Adverse events that require expedited reporting are also recorded in the case report form or other applicable data forms. Special care should be taken to record the event with the same terminology and supporting data as were reported on the SAE report form, unless time has provided different information from what was originally submitted.

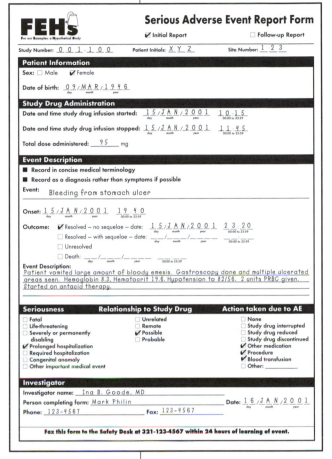

Sponsor Responsibilities

During the Investigational New Drug application phase, the sponsor is responsible for both expedited and routine reporting of adverse events to the FDA. Reporting then continues even after the drug has been approved for marketing.

5. Adverse Events

Expedited Reporting

The sponsor is required to report to the FDA in an expedited manner all adverse events that are:

1 Serious

2 Unexpected (not in investigator's brochure)

3 Study treatment-related

The sponsor must report these events in writing to the FDA within 15 calendar days of first knowledge of the event.

When an event is also fatal or life-threatening in addition to being serious, unexpected, and study-treatment related, the sponsor must report it to the FDA by telephone (or fax) within seven calendar days, followed by a written report within eight additional calendar days.

In order to meet these regulatory requirements of reporting adverse events to the FDA within the appropriate timeframes, the designated drug safety group will review the SAE report form submitted by the site and contact the investigator when additional or supporting data are needed. Follow-up information may be requested for ongoing adverse events.

IND Safety Reports

When an adverse event requires expedited reporting to the FDA, the sponsor generates an IND Safety Report to submit to the FDA. These reports may include, but are not limited to:

- A summary of the event

- The treatment arm the patient received (open-label trials)

- Analysis of similar events that have occurred in this trial and/or in past or present trials

- Comments on the occurrence of the same adverse event with similar therapeutic agents in the same patient population

For example, in a trial studying the use of r-PA (a thrombolytic drug) in acute myocardial infarction patients, the report may include the incidence of occurrence of the same adverse event with t-PA (another thrombolytic drug) in acute myocardial infarction patients.

The site will be provided with a modified version of the IND Safety Report that provides the above information to the sites but without the mandatory FDA/regulatory forms. This report may be referred to as an "investigator alert letter" or "safety letter," or an "alert report" when the report is submitted after drug approval and marketing.

The site investigator must submit the IND Safety Report to the site's IRB. In some cases, after reviewing the IND Safety Report, the IRB may ask that the informed consent form be changed to reflect the new safety information. The sponsor will update the investigator's brochure to reflect the additional event data.

Routine Reporting

In addition to having reported applicable events in an expedited manner, the sponsor must provide the FDA with a semi-annual report that lists study discontinuations due to adverse events, all deaths, and all serious adverse events. Once a New Drug Application is approved, the sponsor is required to submit post-marketing adverse event data

---

IND Safety Report

To: All FEHS Investigators

From: FEHS Sponsor

Re: Protocol # 2468-00 - FEHS For our Example: a Hypothetical Study

Date: February 22, 2001

To assure that all investigators are kept current on safety issues and to comply with all applicable FDA regulations, the following summary of a serious adverse event is being sent to all investigators in the FEHS trial. Although the serious adverse event did not occur in a patient randomized to the investigational study agent, all participating investigators must forward a copy of this report to their IRB/ethical review board. This report should also be filed in your FEHS regulatory binder. Please contact me if you have any questions or require additional information.

Serious Adverse Event Summary

STP is a 76 year old male randomized into the FEHS study on January 29, 2001. The study number assigned was 013-346 and the patient was randomized to placebo. STP has a history of smoking, atrial fibrillation and no history of neurologic events.

Study drug (placebo) was administered intravenously per protocol on January 30, 2001, over a 2 hour period. Aspirin was concomitantly administered as per protocol, 325mg orally, within 1 hour of randomization and daily thereafter. On February 3, 2001, the patient experienced symptoms of stroke. A CT scan was performed and a small hemorrhagic stroke confirmed.

Action Taken with Study Drug

None. Patient was administered placebo and dosing had been completed on January 29.

Relationship to Study Drug

Not likely.

Outcome

Patient's symptoms of slurred speech and mild right hemiparesis have resolved and patient was discharged to home on February 15, 2001. No further follow-up is required.

reports on a quarterly basis for the first 3 years after approval, then on an annual basis.

References

1 21 CFR § 312.84 (a)

2 21 CFR § 312.32 (a)

"The progress of science is often affected more by the frailties of humans and their institutions than by the limitations of scientific measuring devices. The scientific method is only as effective as the humans using it. It does not automatically lead to progress."

—Steven S. Zumdahl

Monitoring

6

Monitoring is a broad concept that relates to the sponsor's regulatory requirement for the oversight of clinical investigations. Monitoring takes on several forms, including on-site monitoring visits, audits, and inspections. *On-site monitoring* visits, performed by "monitors," are conducted to oversee the progress of the trial at the investigative site and ensure that the investigator and IRB meet their regulatory requirements and responsibilities. *Site audits* are performed by the sponsor or a sponsor-designee to ensure that the processes and procedures for conducting the study are properly documented and to review patient data and study records to ensure consistency, in a sense, to "monitor" the monitor, site investigator, and IRB. Site inspections are performed by the FDA to "monitor" the sponsor, monitor, investigator, and IRB, to determine if all groups have met their regulatory requirements and responsibilities. *Site inspections* may include a review of study records, patient data, and processes used to ensure proper evidence and documentation of study procedures and confirmation that standards for Good Clinical Practice were met.

On-Site Monitoring

Purpose of On-Site Monitoring

Clinical trials are monitored to assure that:

1 They are conducted according to the protocol.

2 They are conducted in compliance with the Code of Federal Regulations and Good Clinical Practice guidelines.

3 The resources at the investigative sites are adequate to conduct the trial.

4 The required data are collected and recorded accurately.

The person designated to oversee the progress of a clinical trial at investigative sites is known as the monitor. Depending on the study organization, the monitor may be affiliated with the sponsor, an academic research organization, or a contract research organization, and may have a job title such as Clinical Research Associate (CRA) or Clinical Trial Monitor (CTM).

Types of Monitoring Visits

Monitoring visits can be divided into four basic types depending on their timing and the activities performed. These are *pre-study visits, initiation visits, periodic monitoring visits,* and *close-out visits*.

Pre-Study Visit

A *pre-study visit* takes place after an investigator indicates interest in a specific clinical trial. The purpose of this visit is to determine the site's ability to conduct the study. Before the visit, the investigator should review the protocol and investigator's brochure and sign the confidentiality agreement (if required).

During the visit, the monitor will meet with the principal investigator and study coordinator to verify that they have adequate time to devote to the study, have access to the appropriate patient population, and are not involved with competing clinical trials. The monitor will tour the facility to evaluate its adequacy and determine the availability of project-required equipment. The monitor will also evaluate the appropriateness of the facility for patient enrollment and follow-up, study drug storage, and data form storage.

Regulatory Requirement for Monitoring

Sponsors are responsible for ensuring proper monitoring of the investigation and ensuring that the investigation is conducted in accordance with the general investigational plan and protocols contained in the IND (21 CFR § 312.50) or IDE (21 CFR § 812.40).

A sponsor shall select a monitor qualified by training and experience to monitor the progress of the investigation [21 CFR § 312.53(d) (drugs) and 21 CFR § 812.43(d) (devices)].

Other project-specific requirements, such as access to an ECG laboratory, will be evaluated as well.

Topics for the Pre-Study Visit

During the *pre-study visit*, the monitor should discuss the following:

1. Investigator responsibilities (see Chapter 3) and qualifications (summarized on the investigator's curriculum vitae)

2. Qualifications of other site personnel

3. Study objectives, protocol-required procedures, eligibility criteria, and patient recruitment

4. Institutional Review Board (IRB) and informed consent requirements

5. Anticipated adverse event reporting, source documentation, and record retention

6. Space requirements; availability of a secure area for investigational drug or devices; availability of required equipment

In some cases, the sponsor may allow a pre-study evaluation to be performed over the telephone in lieu of an on-site pre-study visit. The sponsor may approve this approach when, for example, the investigative site is already known to the sponsor or monitor. When this approach is used, an in-person evaluation of the personnel and facilities must be done at the *initiation visit*.

Since the pre-study visit is meant simply to assess the feasibility of conducting the study at the site and determine whether the site can manage protocol-specific requirements, this visit itself does not obligate the investigator or the sponsor to work together on the trial being discussed.

Initiation Visit

Once the investigator has agreed to participate in the study, the regulatory documents have been submitted, and the clinical supplies have been shipped to the site, a study *initiation visit* may be conducted. This visit verifies that the investigator and other site study personnel understand the investigator's obligations (21 CFR § 312 Subpart D), the protocol, and the drug or device being studied.

Since there may be some overlap in the topics discussed at the pre-study visit and the initiation visit, the two visits are sometimes combined. Ideally, the initiation visit is scheduled soon after the arrival of study supplies and just before enrollment begins. In some cases, attendance at an investigator meeting replaces the requirement for an initiation visit. In other cases, the sponsor may require an on-site initiation visit in addition to attendance at the investigator meeting.

During the *initiation visit*, the monitor meets with the investigator, sub-investigators (if applicable), study coordinator, and others related to the study, such as pharmacy and laboratory personnel.

Topics for the Initiation Visit

Some of the topics reviewed at the *pre-study visit* may be reviewed again at the *initiation visit*, but in greater depth. These may include:

1 Study overview, including eligibility criteria, procedures, and access to a suitable patient population

2 Regulations and Good Clinical Practice guidelines, including informed consent requirements, IRB obligations, adverse event reporting, and drug accountability

3 Data forms review including Case Report Forms (CRFs)

4 Regulatory documents and study file organization

If a pre-study visit was not conducted, the monitor will take time during the initiation visit to verify that the study staff have adequate resources and time to dedicate to the study, and confirm that the facility is adequate to conduct the study—e.g., the laboratory is properly certified and suitable space is available for drug, device, or related equipment storage.

Periodic Monitoring Visits

After one or more patients are enrolled in the study, a monitoring visit may be scheduled to evaluate the way the study is being conducted and to perform source document verification. While there is only one pre-study visit or initiation visit conducted per site, there may be numerous *periodic monitoring visits* conducted throughout the trial. The number of visits will be determined by several factors outlined in the monitoring plan, including the number of patients enrolled and the percentage of records that require on-site review, among others.

Topics for Periodic Monitoring Visits

Regardless of how often a monitor visits a site or the amount of data reviewed, each *periodic monitoring visit* is designed to ensure that:

1 the trial is being conducted according to the protocol and that any deviations are appropriately documented;

2 the data on individual data forms/CRFs are accurate and complete when compared with source documents (e.g., medical records, laboratory results, etc.);

3 the patients enrolled met the study eligibility criteria;

4 the principal investigator and other trial personnel are fulfilling their obligations as set forth by the Code of Federal Regulations and the Good Clinical Practice guidelines; and

5 drug accountability procedures are being followed.

Since the monitor has observed how the study is conducted at various other institutions, the monitor may also offer helpful suggestions to facilitate enrollment and protocol adherence. The monitor may be able to share worksheets, educational tools, and additional items created by other investigators and study coordinators that have improved protocol and patient compliance or ensured documentation of protocol-designated data points.

When calling to schedule a *periodic monitoring visit*, the monitor will request that the completed case report forms and serious adverse event forms are available for patients enrolled since the previous monitoring visit. Signed consent forms and hospital and/or outpatient records need to be available for review. The monitor may estimate the amount of time required for this visit based on the anticipated activities and number of forms requiring review.

Preparing for a Monitoring Visit

In preparation for a *periodic monitoring visit*, the investigator and study coordinator should ensure that the following activities have been done prior to the visit. This will ensure a productive monitoring visit for both the monitor and the site study personnel.

1 Identify a quiet place for the monitor to work (an office, conference room, medical records department) that provides access to a telephone, fax, and photocopy machine.

2 Complete the appropriate case report forms prior to the visit.

3 Confirm that Serious Adverse Event (SAE) forms have been submitted and are available for review during the visit.

4 Obtain the medical records and transfer records from outside hospitals, when applicable, for the case report forms identified for review.

5 Organize study file documents for review.

6 Confirm that the signed consent forms for all enrolled patients are available.

7 Schedule an appointment for the monitor to meet with the pharmacist if requested.

8 Schedule time for the study coordinator to meet with the monitor to review all case report forms monitored during the visit and to discuss the general progress of the trial (e.g., enrollment strategies and protocol adherence).

9 Schedule an appointment for the monitor to meet with the investigator to review the findings.

Checking data against source documents, clarifying discrepancies and misinterpretations on the case report forms, and observing and providing practical ideas for implementation of the protocol at specific sites make *periodic monitoring visits* an integral aspect of a successful clinical trial. Refer to the periodic monitoring visit checklist (p. 87) for an example of the activities performed during these visits.

Close-Out Visits

A *close-out visit* may be the last in a series of routine monitoring visits, or it may be scheduled for this purpose

During an on-site **close-out visit,** the monitor may:

- Discuss timelines and strategies for the completion of outstanding case report forms and queries

- Oversee the return or destruction of study drug

- Collect outstanding patient data forms and study forms such as the monitoring and screening logs

- Perform a final review of the study file documents

- Discuss the plans for record retention

once the study has been completed and all case report forms and other pertinent data forms have been submitted.

In some trials, the activities performed to close out a study site are conducted via telephone or written communication rather than during an on-site monitoring visit. When this occurs, sites will be provided with the necessary information and forms to complete this process.

Monitoring Plan

At the beginning of a study, the sponsor determines how monitoring will be performed and who will be responsible for monitoring the trial. Together, the sponsor and monitoring group establish a monitoring plan, which usually includes answers to the following questions:

Will a pre-study visit or initiation visit be required?

When a site and an investigator are known to the sponsor, a *pre-study visit* may not be required. In some trials, an Investigator Meeting that brings together investigators from many sites in one meeting substitutes for an *initiation visit*.

Periodic Monitoring Visit Checklist

1 Patient Status
- ☐ Discuss patient recruitment strategies.
- ☐ Ensure correct randomization procedures and maintenance of study blind.
- ☐ Verify the status of all study patients.

2 Study Supplies Storage/Accountability
- ☐ Ensure that adequate study supplies are available, including study drugs/devices.
- ☐ Ensure the accuracy of receipt and dispensing records.
- ☐ Meet with personnel who dispense study drugs/devices to resolve problems.
- ☐ Inspect storage facilities as appropriate.

3 Regulatory Issues
- ☐ Ensure maintenance of appropriate study files.
- ☐ Ensure continuing IRB notification/reporting as appropriate to include periodic IRB renewals, protocol amendments, and safety reports.
- ☐ Verify that informed consent procedures are being followed and that a consent form is present for each patient.
- ☐ Collect any new or revised regulatory documents.

4 Laboratory Issues
- ☐ Review protocol-specific laboratory requirements.
- ☐ Ensure proper handling of all laboratory specimens.
- ☐ Resolve any problems related to the collection of samples or the performance of local, central, or core laboratories.

5 Responsibilities of Site Study Personnel
- ☐ Review responsibilities of site personnel to determine if changes in personnel or responsibilities have occurred since the last monitoring visit.
- ☐ Provide training for site personnel when needed, including new study personnel, changes in study procedures, or a change in the conduct of the study such as a protocol amendment.

6 Serious Adverse Event (SAE) Status
- ☐ Review SAEs that occurred at the site.
- ☐ Obtain additional SAE information from site as needed.
- ☐ Ensure that all SAEs have been reported accurately and appropriately.

7 Source Document Review/Verification of Data
- ☐ Verify accuracy of CRFs compared to source documents.
- ☐ Review CRFs for incorrect data, omissions, and out-of-range variables.
- ☐ Review source documents for adherence to protocol.
- ☐ Collect original copies of completed CRFs.
- ☐ Generate data queries.
- ☐ Obtain responses to outstanding data queries.

8 Outstanding Issues
- ☐ Determine actions to be taken by the site for outstanding or unresolved issues.
- ☐ Determine actions to be taken by the sponsor for outstanding or unresolved issues.

9 Meet with Investigator and Study Coordinator
- ☐ Discuss overall progress of trial.
- ☐ Discuss new developments affecting patient safety/conduct of trial.
- ☐ Discuss outstanding issues and actions to be taken by the site and/or sponsor.
- ☐ Send a follow-up letter to the investigator.

How frequently will monitoring visits to each site be conducted?

The frequency of monitoring visits will depend on the number of patients enrolled, the number of sites involved, the rate of enrollment, and the volume of source document verification to be performed. Other factors that may affect the frequency of visits as the study progresses are the site's performance and enrollment rate, turnover of site study staff, and problems or concerns related to protocol adherence or patient safety issues. Some of these factors— in particular, the percentage of patient case report forms (CRFs) to be monitored (many trials do not perform 100% monitoring of CRFs)—may be discussed and negotiated with the FDA before the trial is initiated.

What are the responsibilities of the monitors?

Monitors' responsibilities vary from one trial to another. In some trials, the monitor serves as a liaison between the sponsor and the investigative site and is the contact person for all questions ranging from regulatory documents to specific clinical questions about the study. In other trials, the monitor may have only on-site data verification responsibilities, while other personnel are responsible for answering trial-related questions.

How much source document verification will be performed? What percentage of case report forms will be reviewed and compared against source documents at the site?

The amount of on-site source document verification will be based on the type of trial and the phase of the study, among other factors. Some of the options for source document verification are:

1 a review of all data variables in the case report forms of all enrolled patients;

2 a review of all CRF data for a percentage (e.g., 5%) of patients enrolled;

3 a review of only specified variables on all CRFs (e.g., all study endpoint data); and

4 submission of source documents for a review of CRFs in-house (where the data will be entered and reviewed).

Documenting Monitoring Visits

After each monitoring visit, the monitor's findings will be documented, summarized, and discussed with both the investigator and the study coordinator. These findings will be documented in a follow-up letter or progress report, which the site should place in the study file. Any actions taken by the monitor or suggestions to resolve deficiencies will also be included in the follow-up letter/progress report. Any problems should be addressed to the satisfaction of the monitor or sponsor. Monitors also complete a comprehensive site visit report (often called a "trip report") that is submitted to the study sponsor or sponsor-designee.

Whenever a monitor visits a site (except for a *pre-study visit*) the monitor will sign a monitoring log that documents the name of the monitor and the date and purpose of the visit. The monitoring log should be kept in the site's study file.

Sample Follow-up Letter

FEHS
For our Examples: a Hypothetical Study

February 14, 2001

Dear Dr. Candoit,

A monitoring visit for FEHS was conducted at your site on February 12, 2001. During this visit, I reviewed CRFs and associated source documents for 8 of the subjects enrolled at your site. I also reviewed your regulatory documents file and drug accountability records. Your study coordinator was very helpful in answering my questions and worked cooperatively to resolve CRF discrepancies identified through source document verification of the recorded data.

The following issues were identified at this visit:

■ On one patient, baseline laboratory values were not obtained within 24 hours of randomization (patient #6 had results from 28 hours before randomization).

■ A 12-lead ECG was not obtained at discharge on patient #3 as required by protocol.

■ The Investigators' Drug Brochure and a blank copy of your IRB-approved consent form must be placed in your regulatory file.

■ A copy of the drug accountability records must be maintained in the site study file as well as in the investigational pharmacy files.

Your site has done an excellent job of enrolling subjects and performing protocol-required procedures in this trial. The CRFs were completed with a high degree of accuracy and consistency, and all source documents were available for my review.

I thank you and your study coordinator for your time and assistance during this visit. Please call me if you have any questions about the above noted items or any other concerns or questions you may have.

Sincerely,

Your Monitor

Audits and Inspections

In addition to on-site visits by monitors, two other groups may conduct visits at the investigative site. A sponsor may perform an audit, or quality assurance visit, at the site to ensure that proper documentation of processes and procedures are in place and review patient records and data forms, and the FDA may perform either a study-directed or an investigator-directed inspection.

Sponsor Quality Assurance Audits

During or after a trial, auditors from the sponsor (or sponsor designee) may visit selected sites to conduct a quality assurance audit. These inspections ensure that both the monitor and the site study staff are performing their duties according to the Code of Federal Regulations, the protocol, and the site's standard operating procedures. Sponsor audits also help to ensure that future FDA inspections will be uneventful and that the data are suitable for a regulatory submission such as a New Drug Application or a Pre-Market Approval for a device. These visits are much like periodic monitoring visits, and can be viewed by the investigator and study coordinator as an opportunity to improve trial management at their site. Sponsor audits are common practice in clinical drug trials for which an Investigational New Drug (IND) application has been submitted.

A typical inspection lasts from one to two days; the investigator will be given an agenda and a list of data collection forms and documents needed for review, including the study file and IRB records. Case report forms, source documents, the site study file, and signed consent forms may be reviewed, as well as drug/device storage and

Why Audit a Clinical Trial?

- to ensure that the monitors are performing their job accurately;

- to ensure that investigators and staff are performing their jobs appropriately;

- to ensure that future regulatory inspections will be uneventful; and

- to ensure that data for regulatory submission will be suitable.

accountability records. Regulatory documents are typically reviewed to ensure that IRB approval was obtained and documented before initiating the study, that informed consent was obtained before beginning any study procedures, that education and training of applicable personnel was performed and documented, and that proper study agent administration procedures were followed and documented.

Auditors will review study records to ensure that an *audit trail* exists. An audit trail refers to the ability to follow data from the patient, to the data forms, to the data center and sponsor, and through data processing and analysis to the final written report. This is particularly important when data are changed or corrected after the initial submission of data by the investigator. Records must be kept for all original and corrected data, with indication of who made the changes and when the changes were made.

Information from an audit is typically for internal use by the sponsor, and often the site is not given a copy of the audit report. However, the investigator may be informed of the overall results of the audit and whether the trial data are or are not acceptable.

Food and Drug Administration Inspections

The FDA's Bioresearch Monitoring Program was instituted in 1977 as a result of a field program conducted from 1972 to 1974 to determine the compliance of investigational studies. This program indicated a need for the FDA to conduct regular inspections of clinical investigators. The Monitoring Program now regulates inspections of investigators, institutional review boards, sponsors, monitors, contract research organizations, academic research organizations, bioequivalence facilities, and animal testing facilities. The purpose of the program is to

Inspection of Investigator's Records and Reports

An investigator shall upon request permit the FDA (at reasonable times and by properly authorized individuals) to have access to, and copy and verify any records or reports made by the investigator as related to disposition of study drug or device, case histories, and study files. The investigator is not required to divulge subject names unless specific subject records require a more detailed review, or there is reason to believe that the records are incomplete, inaccurate, false, or misleading [Synopsis of 21 CFR § 312.68 and 21 CFR § 812.145].

assure the quality and integrity of the data submitted, to demonstrate the safety and efficacy of regulated products, and to determine that human rights and the welfare of research subjects are protected.

The FDA is authorized by law to inspect clinical sites conducting trials under an IND/IDE at any point during the trial. Inspections can occur even after the investigator has completed participation in the trial and results are submitted.

When an investigator is selected for an inspection, the FDA will contact the investigator, usually by telephone, to arrange a mutually acceptable time for the visit. Sponsors often request that investigators notify them when the site is contacted about an FDA inspection. Sponsors may want to help the site prepare for an FDA inspection to ensure that it runs smoothly.

Upon arrival at the clinical site the inspector will show credentials (photo ID) and present a Form FDA 482, *Notice of Inspection* to the investigator.

The inspection usually begins by determining the facts surrounding the conduct of the study:

1 Who has responsibility for the various activities?

2 What delegation of authority has occurred?

3 Where were specific aspects of the study performed?

4 How and where were data recorded?

5 How was article accountability maintained?

6 How did the monitor communicate with the clinical investigator?

7 How did the monitor evaluate the study's progress?

The FDA inspector has the right to access and copy study records. Data forms are compared with patient records and other source documents that support the data. The inspector may examine patient records that pre-date the study to determine whether the medical condition being studied was properly diagnosed and if an interfering medication was given before the study began. Records covering a reasonable period after completion of the study may also be reviewed to determine if there was proper follow-up and if all signs and symptoms reasonably attributable to the product's use were reported.

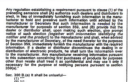

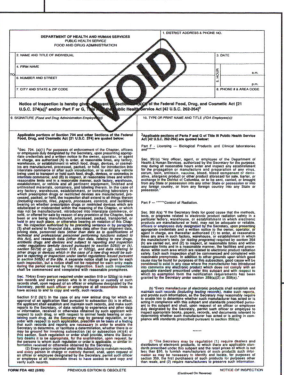

Study-Directed Inspections

Study-directed inspections are conducted for trials that are pivotal to product marketing applications such as New Drug Applications (NDAs), Product License Applications (PLAs) for biological products, and Pre-Market Approval applications (PMAs) for medical devices.

During these visits, the inspector examines data collection forms, giving particular attention to protocol adherence and data integrity. Documentation of informed consent, IRB approval, and continuing review of ongoing studies are also verified.

Investigator-Directed Inspections

This type of inspection is initiated if the sponsor or FDA staff has concerns about an investigator or if there is a complaint from a patient about protection violations. The investigator-directed inspection goes into greater depth than a study-directed inspection, covers more case reports, and may span more than one study.

If an investigator fails in his/her obligations, the FDA can reject the study, disqualify the investigator from participating in additional studies, impose restrictions on carrying out future studies, and in the case of fraud, pursue criminal prosecution. In the future, there may be legislation enacted that allows the FDA to impose fines on investigators who commit violations of informed consent and other important research practices.

Inspection Findings and Reports

The FDA conducts an exit interview at the end of all inspections. At this interview, the inspector discusses the findings of the inspection, clarifies misunderstandings, and may issue the investigator a written Form FDA 483, *Inspectional Observations*, documenting deviations from the Code of Federal Regulations. If the investigator disagrees with any of the findings or believes there was a misunderstanding, the investigator should provide the inspector with an explanation of why the investigator believes the observation is not a violation. The investigator must convey the explanation carefully so as to keep a good, open line of communication with the inspector.

Once the findings have been reviewed and discussed with the investigator, the inspector will submit an *Establishment Inspection Report* to the FDA, where it will be reviewed and assigned a final classification. Written notification of the issues will be submitted to the investigator in the form of one of the following:

■ **NAI** — *No Action Indicated:* No objectionable conditions or practices were found during the inspection (or the objectionable conditions found did not

Sample of an Inspectional Observations Form — 483

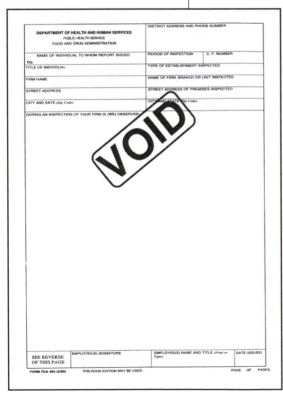

94

justify further action). A letter will be issued that requires no response from the site.

■ **VAI** — *Voluntary Action Indicated:* Objectionable conditions or practices were found, but the FDA is not prepared to take or recommend any administrative or regulatory action. A letter may be issued at the discretion of the FDA depending on the nature of the deviations. This letter may or may not require a response from the investigator; however, if a response is required, the letter will describe what is necessary.

■ **OAI** — *Official Action Indicated:* Regulatory and/or administrative actions will be recommended in a "warning letter" identifying deviations requiring immediate action by the investigator. The FDA may inform both the study sponsor and the site IRB of the deficiencies. They may also inform the sponsor if procedure deficiencies indicate ineffective monitoring by the sponsor.

Investigator Response

The warning letter issued when official action is indicated will specify how quickly the investigator needs to respond, usually within 15 working days. The investigator's response should address each observation and indicate the corrective action taken or the proposal for corrective action including the proposed time period for completion. The tone of the letter should be factual, professional, and cooperative. Depending on the investigator's response, the FDA may require additional follow-up. If the deviations are significant violations of applicable regulations, the FDA can recommend additional sanctions.

"It is one of the most beautiful compensations of life, that no man can sincerely try to help another without helping himself."

—*Ralph Waldo Emerson*

Deciding to be a Principal Investigator

Becoming an investigator in clinical trials has a number of rewards. It can broaden your perspective in the practice of medicine and provides a mechanism for you to participate in testing the newest medical treatments. Participation in clinical trials provides opportunity for interaction with medical science thought leaders in your field and you may be able to participate in authoring publications of study results. Your interactions with enrolled patients may be more in-depth and therefore more satisfying than interactions with other patients in your practice, especially when conducting long-term follow-up trials. These positive outcomes are just some of the benefits that result from the dedicated effort it takes to successfully conduct clinical trials in your office or hospital.

While the positive aspects of being a principal investigator are significant, the responsibilities and accountability are of equal importance and can present the investigator with many challenges. This was recently demonstrated by the tragic death of an 18-year old in a gene-transfer study at the University of Pennsylvania in September 1999. After this young man's death, authorities learned that study subjects in this trial were not adequately protected or fully informed, and that hundreds of adverse events experienced by volunteers enrolled in gene-transfer trials went unreported by investigators.

To bring these issues and concerns to the attention of the research community and highlight steps implemented to correct the problems, Donna Shalala, Secretary of the Department of Health and Human Services (HHS), authored an editorial in the September 14, 2000 issue of *The New England Journal of Medicine*. In the editorial, Shalala describes clinical research trends that have adversely affected the safety of human subjects, and details several steps implemented at the HHS since March 2000.

Two of these trends are that researchers may not be ensuring that subjects fully understand the possible risks and benefits of a study, and that too many researchers do not comply with the standards of good clinical practice. This includes enrolling subjects who do not meet study eligibility criteria, not reporting adverse events as required, not following the protocol, and not training staff adequately. One of the steps to counter these problems will be implementing an aggressive educational and training effort to ensure that all investigators, research administrators, IRB members, and IRB staff have appropriate training in bioethics and other research-related issues involving human subjects.

The emergence of these issues in the public discourse emphasizes that, although involvement in clinical research is a challenging and rewarding experience for many, it is not for everyone. As a potential investigator in clinical trials, you must carefully consider a number of research-related issues that affect this decision. To successfully conduct clinical trials, you must determine if you have the time to perform the oversight required, and if so, evaluate how this research can best be incorporated into your practice.

Personal Motivation and Interests

Health care providers enjoy participating in clinical research for a number of reasons. Among these are the opportunity to stay abreast of the latest treatments in your specialty area, the ability to offer new products to patients, and the opportunity to interact with colleagues involved in clinical trials. In addition, you may be able to enlist the support of others in their hospital or practice to broaden the clinical research opportunities available throughout the institution.

While it is rewarding to be able to offer new treatment opportunities to patients, remember that not all patients participating in clinical trials personally benefit from the investigational drug. Patient benefit may not occur if the patient was given placebo, or a dose that proved to be sub-therapeutic, or if the investigational treatment proved to be ineffective. However, even when patients participating in clinical research do not benefit from the treatment under investigation, most patients do benefit from the increased contact with the investigator and study personnel. Additionally, the knowledge gained from an individual's participation adds to the body of knowledge that contributes to the care of future patients with the same disease process.

Your participation in clinical trials will require a substantial time commitment. While many research-related tasks may be delegated to a study coordinator or subinvestigator, the investigator accepts ultimate responsibility for the study and patient safety. In order to maintain the study integrity, protocol adherence, and reporting requirements, the investigator must remain fully involved and informed throughout the trial.

Adhering to a protocol sometimes requires performing procedures or treating patients differently from clinical practice. While patient safety will of course be foremost in your mind, following the protocol carefully is critical to determining if the new treatment is safe and effective.

Some Investigator Tasks and Time Commitments

- Orienting partners and staff to the protocol

- Adapting office routines (and/or documentation of routines) to the protocol requirements

- Attending investigator meetings

- Screening, enrolling, and consenting patients

- Communicating with site study staff and sponsor (or designee) study personnel

- Performing study-related procedures and follow-up visits

- Reviewing case report forms and other patient data forms

Staffing to Support Clinical Trials

A study site cannot effectively and efficiently participate in clinical trials without sufficient staffing resources. One of the trends adversely affecting clinical research identified by HHS Secretary Shalala, is the failure to adhere to the standards of good clinical practice and to ensure that study personnel are adequately trained. Therefore, not only does your site need an adequate number of personnel, but all personnel must be trained appropriately.

Activities performed by study personnel may vary from one trial to another, depending on many study-specific factors; however, there are personnel needs pertinent to most trials. A study coordinator, sub-investigators, and support personnel can all work closely with you to ensure that the study meets regulatory requirements and good clinical practice standards, including the protection of human subjects and patient confidentiality.

Study Coordinator

In particular, the role of the study coordinator is vital to the success of a trial. Most investigators employ an individual who can work with the investigator to accomplish the detailed tasks required for study implementation. The specific activities delegated to the study coordinator by the investigator vary according to the needs of a particular trial, but for all trials you should discuss these activities with your study coordinator well before the trial begins, and establish a plan for regular communication and review of activities.

You should not underestimate the time required to perform these activities. A common mistake is to assume that these duties can be performed during a lunch break or in addition to other full-time job responsibilities. A part-time study coordinator is a realistic option for some trials and activities, but in order to work effectively the study coordinator should be available during some business hours to see patients, talk with representatives from the sponsor, and perform other study-related tasks.

Some trials have challenging entry criteria that can make screening patients a labor-intensive process. In many trials, protocol adherence and data collection is complex and detailed. If you are aware of these issues and find creative ways to provide incentives to staff who devote significant time and effort to a trial, you can help prevent staff burnout. Incentives can be as grand as providing transportation to a professional meeting or establishing an education grant, or as simple as a lunch or trial tee-shirt. If your staff remains enthusiastic about a study, patient enrollment and follow-up will benefit. The work performed early in a study (preparation of materials for IRB review, orientation of site staff, development of data worksheets, etc.) will often pay off in increased enrollment, while the work performed throughout the remainder of the study (completing data forms, reporting adverse events, patient follow-up, etc.) will result in accurate and complete patient data. A well-motivated staff can make this happen.

While the study coordinator is often a registered nurse, a nursing background is not a requirement. Study coordinators can come from a variety of backgrounds, but should have some knowledge of medicine, disease conditions, and how to interact with patients. The following traits or qualities are found in most successful study coordinators.

1 *Attention to detail.* This is required in most aspects of clinical trial work. Examples of detail work include

performing protocol-required procedures and tests that need to be completed in a designated manner at specific timepoints, completing patient data forms, and dispensing study drug and completing accountability documents.

2 *Good communication skills.* Study coordinators interact with people of varied backgrounds and educational levels who are involved in all aspects of the trial, including the sponsor, monitors, site study staff, laboratory personnel, study personnel at other sites, and patients. Your study coordinator must also communicate effectively with you throughout the course of the study. Training skills and the ability to convey and generate enthusiasm when teaching other site personnel about the studies are also important.

3 *Flexibility.* A successful study coordinator moves quickly from one task to another and handles a workload that may change daily. The study coordinator may be completing paperwork to submit to the IRB on one day, and conducting outpatient visits and processing blood samples for another study the next day. The ability to oversee multiple tasks simultaneously and set priorities is important.

4 *Ability to work independently.* The investigator should clearly delineate the study coordinator's responsibilities and expectations. An effective study coordinator will be able to take this information and function independently without your direct oversight of each activity.

5 *Organizational skills.* The study coordinator has many tasks to juggle at once; thus, the ability to manage numerous activities and work well under pressure is essential. There are many deadlines to meet, including IRB submissions and data form completion, and tasks (such as reporting serious adverse events) that must be handled within specified time frames.

Sub-investigators

When a trial requires a significant amount of physician time—for example, to obtain informed consent, perform physical assessments, or conduct outpatient visits—it may be helpful to identify individuals who can function as sub-investigators. Sub-investigators must be listed in section 6 on the Form FDA 1572 (for trials conducted under an Investigational New Drug application) as individuals who will be assisting the investigator in the conduct of the clinical trial. While you may delegate some duties to sub-investigators, it remains your responsibility to ensure that the study is conducted according to the protocol regardless of who performs study-specific activities.

Support Personnel

It is often important to have support personnel on the clinical trial team who can perform tasks such as photocopying, faxing, and scheduling appointments. This will allow all study personnel to best use their time and skills.

Space and Resource Needs

Your site may need additional space and resources when participating in clinical trials. Some of these will be necessary for all trials while others are study-specific. The following needs are similar for most trials; therefore, plan to address these needs before taking on your first trial.

Workspace for Study Coordinator

A quiet workspace with a desk and telephone is needed for the study coordinator, who is required to make frequent telephone calls and complete a variety of data forms. Ideally, the study coordinator's workspace has room for the locked file cabinets needed to store patient data forms, and is near the location where patients are evaluated or treated in the study. This location allows trial data forms and study reference materials to be readily available during patient visits.

Equipment

Access to photocopy and fax machines is also necessary. A computer may be needed to retrieve patient data and reports and, increasingly, is needed for entering data collected during the study. In addition, some studies are now using the Internet to disseminate and retrieve study materials.

Storage Space

You'll need storage space for patient data collection forms and study files. Depending on the trial, patient study files may need to be kept for as long as 15 years. In trials where study drug is stored in the office of the study coordinator or the investigator rather than in the pharmacy, secure storage must be available. Only study-related personnel should have access to study drug, study records, and patient files.

Additional Space

Availability of a quiet work area is necessary for individuals monitoring the trial, to review patient and study records and meet with the study coordinator. A conference room or an unoccupied office can often be used for this purpose.

Your Local Institutional Review Board

Familiarity with your local Institutional Review Board (IRB) and its policies and procedures is key to the success of a clinical trial. Identify where and to whom the protocol and applicable study documents should be submitted, the frequency and time of IRB meetings, and the deadlines for submitting a protocol in order to ensure its review at the next scheduled meeting. The frequency with which IRBs meet varies from one institution to another, and ranges from weekly to monthly and even bimonthly or quarterly meetings. It may be necessary to submit the protocol and associated documents a week or more before the meeting, allowing IRB members adequate time to review the protocol and prepare for the meeting.

If there is not an IRB at your site, an IRB external to your site can review and approve your clinical trial protocols. These external IRBs are often referred to as "central IRBs" and are commercial enterprises that will review and approve protocols for many investigators at different institutions. Centralized IRBs can offer efficient service to clinical sites because IRB members performing this work full-time are thoroughly familiar with the protocol when reviewing the same protocol for multiple sites. Central IRBs charge a fee for their services that may vary with different protocols.

One of the challenges facing external IRBs located outside the community is fulfilling the regulatory requirement for "sensitivity to local factors." Local laws, institutional policies, professional and community standards, and population differences are all local factors that an IRB must consider when reviewing a protocol. A centralized review must allow for these important differences from one investigative site to another, based on the surrounding community and population.

Another option for obtaining IRB review and approval of a protocol is to determine if there is an IRB outside your institution that has unique expertise in your area of interest. The IRB of a large local hospital or tertiary care center may function in this role. This IRB may be willing to review protocols from nearby sites, with a representative from each site present at the meetings. This system helps overcome concerns about local factors. You may also be able to share an IRB with another nearby institution. In this case, both sites would contribute to the IRB membership and to the responsibility for reviewing protocols from the two institutions.

Establishing an IRB

When no IRB exists at your site, one option is to establish your own. Talk to people within your institution to consider the options available and determine if there is sufficient interest and support for establishing an on-site IRB. Try contacting the IRB of another local institution that is willing to offer operational advice on establishing a new IRB within a site. Refer to the regulations pertaining to IRBs in Part 56 of Title 21 of the Code of Federal Regulations to ensure that the newly established IRB complies with all regulations (see Appendix C).

Examples of Local Factors

- A Catholic hospital may have a requirement that protocols and consent forms not make reference to birth control.

- The city of Seattle, Washington, requires that individuals participate in state counseling before enrolling in an AIDS trial.

"Let no act be done at haphazard, nor otherwise than according to the finished rules that govern its kind."

—*Marcus Aurelius Antoninus,* Meditations

The Protocol

8

Study Procedure Implementation at the Site

In some situations, site staffing or personnel issues dictate how study-required procedures will be implemented. For example, one site may have hospital laboratory personnel available to obtain protocol-required blood samples and perform the centrifuging, labeling, and freezing of the specimens, while at another site the study coordinator may be responsible for these tasks.

In other situations, logistical issues at the site may determine how protocol-related procedures can be completed. For example, in a study where patients are enrolled in the emergency department and must receive study drug within a very short time after study randomization, a hospital with a 24-hour pharmacy near the emergency department may store study drug in the pharmacy. However, an institution without a convenient pharmacy or 24-hour pharmacy staff may require study drug to be stored in a secure location within the emergency department.

The protocol is the document that provides the background and framework for the planned study and describes how the study will be implemented. Protocol authors often solicit the input of thought leaders and clinicians practicing in the field to ensure the protocol is statistically sound enough to meet its stated objectives, is practical for sites to enroll patients, and can be completed in the proposed time frame. Many trials have a Steering Committee (a group of experts in the area of study) responsible for the oversight of a proposed trial or group of trials. Steering Committee members often contribute to protocol design, including clinical issues, subject safety, and statistical matters.

Protocols are written by trial sponsor personnel, individual investigators, clinicians, scientists, or any combination of these individuals. The sponsor submits the final protocol to the FDA as part of an Investigational New Drug application or Investigational Device Exemption application for approval before initiating clinical trials. The protocol must also be approved by each investigative site's Institutional Review Board (IRB) before study enrollment at the specific site can begin.

Protocols vary greatly in writing style, content, and flow, but should provide the individual investigator with a thorough understanding of the goals of the study and the procedures involved. Depending on the written discussion of the background work and previous trials conducted, the complexity of the trial, required procedures, and many other factors, protocols may range in length from one or two pages to more than 100 pages, with 40–60 pages being a typical length.

Once a protocol is finalized and approved by the FDA, it becomes the final authority on enrollment criteria and study procedures. While investigative sites may employ site-specific methods when implementing the study, specific eligibility criteria and study-required procedur must be followed carefully. If changes to the protocol are indicated after initial FDA approval is obtained, the authors write a correction or addition (known as an amendment) and submit it to the FDA. Once the FDA approves the protocol amendment, it must be submitted to and approved by the IRB at each site as well.

The first part of this chapter provides a brief overview of the common components of a protocol, while the latter part of the chapter identifies many questions that should be answered when reviewing a specific protocol.

Common Components of a Protocol

Protocols come in many styles and sizes depending on the study phase, the type of product under investigation, and many other factors. In addition to collecting data in an effort to answer the question put forth, the protocol design must also ensure that regulatory requirements are met, including informed consent, reporting of adverse events, and protocol adherence.

Background and Rationale

The background section of the protocol describes the results of pre-clinical studies and previous clinical trials. Adequate information pertaining to safety and efficacy demonstrated in previous studies should be provided. The rationale for the study should clearly state the reason why it is being conducted based on the background information provided.

Sample Table of Contents for a Protocol

I.   Introduction
        a. Background
        b. Rationale

II.   Objectives

III.   Trial Design
        a. Patient Selection
        b. Randomization
        c. Treatment Plan

IV.   Schedule of Assessments

V.   Study Drug
        a. Preparation, Packaging, and Labeling
        b. Dosing Schedule
        c. Storage, Dispensing, and Disposal/Return
        d. Accountability Records

VI.   Data Collection

VII.   Adverse Event Reporting

VIII.   Statistical Analysis

IX.   Ethical Considerations
        a. Informed Consent
        b. Confidentiality

X.   Monitoring

XI.   Publication of Results

8. The Protocol

Objectives/Endpoints

The objectives of the study are often stated as primary and secondary endpoints (variables). Endpoints are measures believed to quantify the potential effect of a treatment or therapy under study. In addition to clinical endpoints, quality-of-life and economic factors may also be identified as endpoints.

Endpoints should be:

1 Clinically relevant

2 Objective

3 Likely to be affected by the treatment under investigation

The study of quality-of-life is a growing field in which issues that have an impact on one's physical abilities (physiological function), psychological function, well-being (spiritual function), and social functioning are evaluated. A number of validated instruments have been used to evaluate aspects of quality-of-life based on patient responses. Some quality-of-life instruments measure generic health status while others are disease-specific.

With cost containment and health care reform, answering questions related to the short- and long-term costs of treatment has become increasingly important. The economic impact of a treatment can be measured in terms of direct and indirect costs. Direct costs include the actual charges for hospitalization, treatment, drugs, medical supplies, and professional services; these are listed on a patient's bill. Indirect costs are more difficult to measure and include such things as time away from work, loss of wages, and pain and suffering.

Examples of Endpoints

- Death
- Stroke
- Rehospitalization
- Quality-of-life parameters
- Economic factors
- Tumor regression/tumor size

Study Design

The design of a study functions as the framework by which the study objectives will be met. Many factors are considered when determining the design for a given trial, including the use of control groups, randomization strategies, and whether a study can or should be blinded to investigators and/or study subjects. While they are not always feasible to design as such, randomized, double-blind, placebo-controlled trials are considered the "gold standard" of clinical trial design.

Use of Control Groups

When the makeup of the groups of subjects being evaluated is controlled, it creates more homogenous groups for comparison. Thus investigators can conclude that differences in the groups are related to the treatment under investigation, rather than to differences within the groups. Examples of types of controls include use of placebo, use of active medication, no-treatment, administration of a different dose of the same medicine, and treatment with current standard care. When no standard treatment exists, some control groups will be given no treatment, while other control groups may be given a placebo (inert substance) to serve as the "control."

Randomization

Randomization is the technique of assigning patients to treatment groups without bias. The goal of randomization is to produce treatment groups that are as similar as possible, so that the differences seen in patient outcomes reflect the effect of the treatment rather than differences in the treatment groups themselves. In spite of the implied meaning of the term "random," there is usually nothing random about the planning and strategies used in determining the type of randomization employed in a study. The randomization scheme is typically developed by

Examples of Quality-of-Life Instruments

The SF-36, one of the most frequently used instruments to measure health-status, is made up of 36 questions covering eight domains:

1. Physical functioning

2. Role limitations due to physical health problems

3. Bodily pain

4. General health

5. Vitality

6. Social functioning

7. Role limitations due to emotional problems

8. Mental health

The WOMAC (Western Ontario and McMasters University Osteoarthritis Index) instrument is a disease-specific measure of health status designed for use in osteoarthritis studies. Its use allows researchers to measure the intensity of pain and frustration of functional limitations related to arthritis.

The FACT-G is a 27-item questionnaire focusing on physical wellbeing, social/family wellbeing, emotional wellbeing, and functional wellbeing. This tool is available in 30 different languages and has several different subscales available.

When first used in human subjects in the early 1930s, randomization was accomplished by literally tossing a coin to determine the treatment group assignment. Current methods of randomization vary widely depending on trial design, but include simple randomization (patients assigned treatment based on a code — often by order of admission into the study), block randomization (patients proportionately assigned to treatment groups within a pre-specified number or "block" of subjects), and stratification (patients assigned to treatment groups based on sex, age, weight, intensity of disease, or other relevant prognostic variables expected to affect outcome).

a statistician, taking into account all the relevant aspects of the study design.

Blinding

Blinding is another technique used to avoid introducing bias in a clinical trial. Blinding is the term used for masking the intervention a patient receives in order to reduce bias on the part of the patient or study personnel.

A *single-blind* study is one in which the intervention is unknown to the patient (the patient is "blind" to the treatment). Blinding the patient to treatment reduces the potential for the "placebo effect," the effect seen when a patient believes a beneficial effect has occurred based on the patient's *expectation* of study treatment, rather than on the actual treatment itself. The placebo effect is less likely to occur if the patient is blinded to the treatment.

To prevent investigators and study staff from consciously or unconsciously introducing bias into the study, study drug may be double-blinded. A *double-blind* study is one in which both the study participants and those administering the study drug (the investigator and study staff) are "blinded" to the treatment being given.

Double-dummy is a technique used to maintain the blind when two treatments cannot be manufactured to appear identical. Supplies are prepared for "treatment A" (active drug A and identical placebo A) and for "treatment B" (active drug B and identical placebo B). Subjects take one from each treatment set of drugs — either active drug A and placebo B or active drug B and placebo A.

Unblinding. When knowledge of the study assignment is needed to determine the appropriate treatment of unexpected events that occur in a study patient, unblinding is necessary. The criteria and process for unblinding should be described in the protocol even though it is expected to occur only rarely.

It is not always possible, however, to provide for blinding in a study. In some studies, it may be impossible to blind the people who administer a medicine or treatment (for example, giving a nebulized treatment versus chest percussion therapy), or when subjects are randomized to device implantation versus no device.

Study Population

The protocol describes the target population in terms of eligibility as divided into inclusion and exclusion criteria. These criteria typically relate to patient characteristics, characteristics of the disease and treatment, the results of screening tests, and other factors. Eligibility criteria often refer to patient age, pre-existing history and conditions, reproductive capability, and screening laboratory values in addition to the specific disease or condition being treated.

The protocol usually identifies how many subjects will be enrolled over a specific period of time, and may note the number of sites and countries participating in the study. As a general rule, subjects should not participate in more than one trial at a time; however, there are exceptions to this. The protocol should identify whether subjects may participate in concurrent studies or specify the time period that must elapse since last participating in another trial.

Study Treatment Plan

The protocol should clearly delineate the activities to be performed in the implementation of the study. This includes a plan for administration of the study treatment and a list of the assessments and procedures that should be performed throughout the duration of the study. Protocols often include a *schedule of assessments*, a chart that lists all study-required assessments and the timepoints at which they should be performed. Required assessments will vary widely depending on the treatment and type of study, and

Common Eligibility Requirements: Inclusion and Exclusion Criteria

Patient Characteristics: sex; age; weight; pregnancy; use/abuse of tobacco, alcohol, and drugs; surgical history; allergy/sensitivity to study drug

Disease and Treatment Characteristics: disease being studied; use of concomitant medications; history of other diseases and hospitalizations; current clinical status

Screening Tests: results of tests or evaluations that would include or exclude a subject from participating

Other Factors: participation in another clinical trial, ability of patient to fully cooperate, geographic location[1]

may include laboratory samples, tests, procedures, examinations, and questionnaires.

Sample Schedule of Assessments					
	Screening/ Baseline	30-Day	90-Day	Major/Minor Bleeding	(Re)MI or Recurrent Ischemia	2 Weeks After Study Drug Stopped
ECG (12-lead)	X				X	X
Vital signs/weight	X					X
Serum pregnancy test	X					
CK-MB and troponin	X				X	
PLT count/Hgb/Hct	X	X	X	X		X
Serum creatinine	X	X	X	X	X	X
WBC, SGPT total bilirubin	X	X	X			X

Safety Assessment, Management, and Reporting

While some safety concerns may be anticipated based on previous studies or the treatment's mechanism of action, the protocol should specify how all safety issues, both expected and unexpected, should be handled. Management of adverse events and reporting requirements should be provided, including the requirements and process for the expedited reporting of events.

Criteria for making changes in the proposed study treatment plan, such as study drug dose increases or reductions, termination, or early withdrawal, should be described in the protocol.

Statistical Aspects

The role of statistics in designing a study and analyzing the results is of critical importance. The trial must be designed to allow appropriate analysis and interpretation of the data. Some of the statistical considerations are listed below.

Sample Size

Sample size refers to the number of patients who complete a trial; sample size must be sufficient to detect the effects of the treatment(s) under investigation in the target population. The number of study subjects should be large enough to provide a reliable answer to the questions being addressed in the protocol and is usually determined by the primary objective(s) of the study. Statistical formulas are used to calculate the number of patients needed to attain a pre-specified event rate. Other issues such as patients who are lost-to-follow-up or noncompliant, and subjects who drop out before study completion must be taken into consideration to determine adequate sample size.

Sample size adjustment may occur in long-term trials when there is an opportunity to check the assumptions upon which the initial sample size calculation was made. An interim check on blinded data may reveal that overall response variances, event rates, or survival is not as anticipated. A sample size adjustment can be calculated if necessary and included in a protocol amendment.

Power

Power represents the ability to detect a statistical difference between treatments when a difference actually exists. Typically, trials are powered to provide at least an 80% chance of detecting a difference.

Trial Statisticians Make Sample Size Calculations Based on:

1 The magnitude of the expected or desired effect

2 The variability (may be estimated) of the events or endpoints being analyzed

3 The desired probability (power) to see the effect with a defined significance level—usually a power of 80% or greater

8. The Protocol

Intention-to-Treat Principle

The intention-to-treat principle has become a standard method of analyzing data in clinical trials. The primary basis of this principle is that treatment effect is best assessed when analyzed as part of the group to which the patient was randomized (intended), no matter what treatment the patient actually received. This means that if a patient received a treatment different from the one to which he was randomized, the data will be analyzed as if the patient received the originally intended treatment. Although the advantages of this principle may not be intuitively obvious, years of theoretical and practical work have demonstrated this type of analysis best in preventing biases from influencing the interpretation of the outcome of a clinical trial.

While exclusion of these individuals from efficacy analyses may seem reasonable, it often led to excluding a large number of enrolled subjects. Exclusion of these patients opposes the purpose of the study—to evaluate the treatment under investigation in patients suspected of meeting the criteria for the target population. In reality, practicing clinicians treat patients prospectively, often based on the disease or condition the patient is suspected of having. Therefore, when analyzing data using the intention-to-treat principle and including all enrolled patients, study findings should more closely resemble the results that will be seen in clinical practice.

Most major trials use the intention-to-treat methodology, although additional analyses evaluating only those patients who received treatment may also be performed. Therefore investigators must be comfortable with all treatment strategies used in a trial and every effort must be made to administer the assigned treatment and ensure that patients receive the full course of study therapy.

Interim Analysis

An interim analysis is one that is performed at any time before the final data analysis, usually to evaluate treatment differences, efficacy, and significant safety issues in Phase IIb and Phase III trials. Interim analyses may be performed for a number of reasons, including ethical and scientific reasons, financial reasons, and practical considerations. Ethical and scientific reasons relate to ensuring that a superior treatment is not withheld from patients longer than necessary; financial concerns relate to the high cost of trials and the expense of continuing a trial that cannot demonstrate significant treatment differences; practical considerations relate to ensuring that a trial is progressing as planned.[2]

The purpose and timing of planned interim analyses must be stated in the protocol. One or more analyses may be specified at designated timepoints during the course of a study. The timing of the interim analyses may be based on enrollment (such as when half of the patients are enrolled), or based on a period of time (for example, 6 months into a year-long enrollment period). The timing and number of interim analyses will vary depending on the study, but are usually planned to represent a cross section of the total enrollment. Since an unplanned interim analysis may flaw the results of a study and weaken the

Example of How the Intention-to-Treat Principle Might Be Applied

A blinded trial is being conducted to compare heparin to an investigational anticoagulant in patients having an acute myocardial infarction. An acutely ill patient is randomized to double-blind study treatment (heparin or investigational anticoagulant). However, after randomization, the clinician decides to give open-label heparin instead of blinded study drug so as to be sure of which treatment the patient is receiving. If the data are analyzed according to actual treatment administered, there would be potential for the group of patients receiving heparin to include more high-risk patients resulting in a bias toward higher mortality in the heparin group. However, if the analysis is performed based on the intention-to-treat principle, the data would be analyzed according to randomization assignment rather than on actual treatment administered. This would keep the treatment groups similar and reduce this type of bias.

Examples of Interim Analysis Findings and Resulting Outcomes or Actions	
Finding	**Outcome or Action**
No significant difference or safety concerns in treatment groups	Continue study as planned
Unequivocal positive effect in one of the treatment groups	Stop study so that all patients can be offered superior treatment
Serious safety concerns with one or more treatment group	Stop or modify study
Lower-than-expected event rate	Increase the number of subjects to be enrolled

confidence in study conclusion, the plan for interim analyses must be carefully thought out and clearly specified in the protocol. The timing and criteria for analysis should be documented, as should guidelines for early termination of the study.

The interim data analysis is performed by a statistician who provides the information to members of a Data and Safety Monitoring Board (see below). Since an interim analysis may require unblinding of treatment group assignments, it should be a completely confidential process. All data presented and reviewed during interim analyses should remain confidential until enrollment has stopped and the trial is unblinded.

Data and Safety Monitoring Board

A Data and Safety Monitoring Board (DSMB) is an independent committee of clinicians, statisticians, ethicists, and other specialists who are knowledgeable in the area of study. This committee is established by the sponsor; the committee membership and responsibilities should be described in the protocol. Other names for this committee include a *Safety and Efficacy Monitoring Committee* (SEMC), *Data and Safety Monitoring Committee* (DSMC), and *Data Monitoring Committee* (DMC). The role of the committee is to assess the progress of a trial, its safety, and its efficacy at specified intervals. The committee may recommend that a study be continued, modified, or stopped based on the data provided at the time of an interim analysis.

Typically, the members of the committee have no involvement in the study nor any financial links to the treatment(s) under study. This is intended to ensure confidentiality and protect the integrity of the data, providing a fair and unbiased review. However, in some Phase II trials, committee members may be representatives from the study sponsor because of their knowledge of the study treatment.

Data Forms and Record Retention

The protocol may identify or include copies of data forms such as the case report form, and outline the timeline for completion and submission of data forms. The length of time for record retention should be provided, as well as the persons to contact before destroying study records at the end of the record retention period.

Monitoring

Monitoring is performed in clinical research to oversee the quality of the trial and the study conduct at the sites where patients are enrolled and treated. Site monitoring typically includes a determination of protocol adherence and source document verification to confirm the accuracy of the data being submitted. The protocol may identify the monitoring plan and may outline the frequency of monitoring visits, the percentage of data forms to be monitored, and the group responsible for the monitoring activities, as well as other aspects of monitoring. Refer to Chapter 6 for more information about monitoring visits.

Reviewing a Specific Protocol

Unless you are involved in the process of developing or finalizing a protocol, you will receive a close-to-final draft or an FDA-approved protocol to review, with the study design and analysis plan already established. When you receive a protocol, you will need to decide if the goals and design of the protocol fit within the scope of your clinical practice.

You will need to carefully review and evaluate how the protocol may be different from your routine clinical practice, determine if the appropriate patient population and resources are available at your institution, and identify whether any investigative site needs that are unique to the protocol can be met at your site.

The following questions will help you determine if participation in a particular study is right for your institution.

Study Design

What type of study is outlined in the protocol? For example, studies may be performed at only one site or at many sites (multi-center), or study drug may be open-label, single-blind, or double-blind with a placebo-control group. In addition to identifying the type of study, consider the following:

1 How do the protocol requirements compare to the routine standard of care for this patient population?

2 Are there non-routine tests or procedures that need to be performed?

3 How long will study enrollment and follow-up last?

4 Are outpatient visits required? How many?

Patient Population

What is the target patient population specified in the protocol, and does your practice or institution see enough patients with the target disease or condition? Because of protocol exclusion criteria, only a small portion of the

patients with the target disease or condition may be
eligible for enrollment.

1 What are the eligibility criteria, and are they broad
enough to allow enrollment of a sufficient number of
patients?

2 How many patients are you expected to enroll, and over
what time period?

3 Is the protocol diagnosis a seasonal condition (e.g.,
asthma, allergic rhinitis) that will limit the time,
number, or frequency of subjects seeking medical care
at the time the study is being conducted?

4 Will physician colleagues participate in the screening of
patients contributing to the number of patients enrolled
at the site?

5 Are there competing clinical trials that target the same
patient population?

Investigator Time Requirements

It is important to quantify the amount of time you need to
oversee patient safety and study staff activities and perform
all study activities within the regulatory requirements and
standards of good clinical practice.

1 Is there a "start-up" meeting, often called an
Investigators' Meeting, which the investigator and study
coordinator should attend? How long does the meeting
last (often one or two days)? Depending on the meeting
length and location, travel to and from the meeting
may be completed in one day, or an overnight stay may
be necessary.

2 How will subjects/patients be recruited? What is the
screening process for patients—are patients easily
identified or will medical charts need to be reviewed to
identify patients?

3 How much time will be required to perform protocol-related activities? For example, if the protocol requires enrollment of five patients per month and patients must be seen every two weeks for approximately 15 minutes per visit, then 2.5 hours of investigator time per month must be set aside to meet with study patients. An additional 3–4 hours per month should be allocated for performing other aspects of the study (e.g., meeting with the study coordinator to review study progress and answer questions, reading study updates, reviewing and signing required forms, and meeting with the monitor during periodic site visits). In this example, an average of 6 hours per month of investigator time should be allocated to the study.

Study Personnel

A review of the protocol will help determine the tasks that can be delegated to study personnel and determine if there are requirements for time, skills, and/or personnel in addition to those already on the clinical research staff.

Study Coordinator

In order to evaluate the work required, estimate the amount of time required to perform each of the protocol-related activities.

1 How many groups of personnel will need to have educational inservices conducted by the study coordinator? Are patients found in the acute care setting, requiring inservicing on all shifts? Are patients found on more than one unit in the hospital? Do laboratory personnel or other technicians need to be made aware of protocol requirements? Will pharmacy personnel need to be inserviced?

2 Where in the hospital are the typical patients with this disease process located? Is it a cardiology patient who

may be found on one or two units in the hospital or a hematology patient who may be on any medical or surgical unit? How long will it take for the study coordinator to screen a typical patient?

3 Will the study coordinator be responsible for preparing or administering the study drug, or will other hospital staff administer study drug?

4 Will the patient require any additional procedures or interventions after receiving study drug? Do vital signs need to be recorded or blood samples drawn? Will the study coordinator or other staff members perform these activities?

5 Do outpatient or follow-up visits need to be conducted? If so, how many and at what time intervals? Will the study coordinator need to schedule the visits and appropriate tests? How much time will the typical visit require of the study coordinator?

6 How many pages are in the patient case report form? Approximately how long will it take to complete? Are most of the data that need to be collected routinely documented in the patient chart, or will worksheets be required to collect data? Will data need to be obtained from transfer hospitals?

7 How frequently will on-site monitoring visits be conducted? The study coordinator may need to allocate 6–8 hours for each monitoring visit.

Support Staff

Depending on the type of study, the amount of paper work, and the scheduling of patients and procedures involved, support staff are usually needed to perform administrative duties and assist the site study team.

1 Are there administrative duties, such as the scheduling of patients or procedures, that can be managed by support staff?

2 If medical records need to be requested and/or photocopied, can this be done by support staff?

Pharmacist

Some institution policies require a pharmacist to handle all investigational drugs while this is not the case at other institutions. Some studies require the participation of a pharmacist, for example, to prepare intravenous study drug in order to maintain the study blind.

1 Will study drug need to be prepared by a pharmacist?

2 Does the protocol require that study drug be stored and dispensed from the pharmacy?

3 If refrigeration is required, is there adequate locked, limited access to refrigerated storage for the study drug?

4 Will the pharmacist maintain the drug accountability records?

Laboratory Tests and Procedures

Will a local or central laboratory, or both, be used for analysis of specimens? How many samples will need to be drawn, and at what time intervals?

1 Are these protocol-required laboratory tests normally performed at the investigative site? Will laboratory personnel need to be trained to process and label specimens? Are there drug levels or other specialized tests that need to be sent to a central core lab, requiring special handling and shipment of samples?

2 Do the laboratory samples require special handling (e.g., -70°C freezer storage or cold centrifuge) that is not available? Will the sponsor provide any of the equipment if not already at your site?

3 If specimens are to be stored and then shipped in batches, is adequate storage available until the shipment date?

4 Are there special shipping or handling instructions, such as dry ice or special containers? Are these provided by the sponsor or available within your institution?

5 Are there procedures that require the cooperation of other departments at the site? Do the personnel in the other departments need to be trained?

6 Are there other central or "core" laboratories that require shipment of patient data? For example, is there an electrocardiogram (ECG) core lab to which all ECGs must be sent for interpretation or an x-ray core lab to which all films must be sent?

Additional Space and Equipment

All clinical trials require some space and equipment dedicated to conducting the study. These needs include shelf or file cabinet space to store study files, patient binders, and other study materials; documents will require long-term storage at the time of study completion. Equipment such as a computer and telephone, and access to a facsimile machine and photocopier are often absolute requirements. However, a specific protocol may require storage, space, or specific modes of communication in addition to those already available. If the available space and equipment at your site are not sufficient to meet the requirements of the trial, determine if the additional resources can be obtained from the sponsor (or other sources).

1 Will the study supplies (data forms and regulatory files) need to be stored for a longer period of time than usual and require more office and/or storage space? Is there

secure space within the institution or at an off-site location for long-term storage of study documents?

2 Is remote data entry via computer required for the study? Will the sponsor supply the computer? Is there adequate workspace for the computer and access to a modem to dial into the database?

3 Will study drug be stored in the office of the study coordinator or investigator? If so, is there adequate locked storage space available for the study drug?

Budget Considerations

It is important to determine the amount of reimbursement from the sponsor and how the payments will be made throughout the course of the study. The reimbursement plan may affect your site's ability to participate in the study, although there are ways to minimize expenses, and high enrollment may help offset costs. Some of the questions that pertain to the study site agreement or contractual agreement with the study sponsor are:

1 If there are IRB submission fees, will the sponsor cover the cost?

2 Will the sponsor provide money to cover the cost of personnel time to prepare for study start-up and enrollment?

3 How often will site payments occur? What milestones (such as randomization, patient visits, completion of case report forms, completion of follow-up, query-clean data) must a site reach to generate a payment?

4 Will the sponsor pay for patients who are screened but determined not eligible for enrollment?

5 Are payments prorated when a patient drops out early?

Payment plans may be arranged in installments with defined timepoints when payments are issued. For example, 10% of the overall study payment may be made when all regulatory documents are submitted and the contract is signed. An additional 60% may be paid when all the patients are enrolled at a site. The last 30% may be paid when all patients have completed their final visits and all patient data forms have been submitted and queried.

Preparing a Budget

A clinical trial budget will help you determine if a specific protocol is economically feasible. The budget should include patient charges for protocol-required tests and procedures, study personnel costs, and institution charges, plus all other applicable costs. A final budget containing the site's actual costs can then be compared to the reimbursement amount that would be received from the sponsor.

Patient Charges

Review the protocol to identify tests and procedures required of patients participating in the study. The *schedule of assessments* provided with the protocol is a good tool to use to list all procedures. Be sure to separate out patient procedures and/or tests that are considered standard treatment that will be performed in the target patient population regardless of participation in the study. When tests and procedures are considered standard treatment, the costs should not be included in the study budget since they will be billed to the patient's insurance carrier. Once the protocol-required procedures and tests have been identified, the next step is to determine the costs associated with each task. A good resource to determine actual costs is the institution's billing or accounting department.

Personnel Costs

In order to develop an accurate budget, a careful review of the protocol will reveal procedures and tasks that will be required of the investigator and study personnel

After the costs of required tests and procedures have been obtained, identify areas where fees may be negotiated. Is the laboratory willing to process samples at a reduced "research" rate? Are your colleagues willing to waive or reduce professional fees for research-related consults? Does the pharmacy have a reduced fee for research-related prescriptions? Once the costs for each test and procedure have been finalized, multiply the cost of each item by the number of times each will be performed. This provides the total cost of a patient's participation in the study.

throughout the trial, including study start-up and close-out. Be certain to evaluate carefully all aspects of a trial that will affect personnel time requirements. For example, an inpatient trial may require more study coordinator time than an outpatient trial because of the time required for daily rounding on enrolled patients and discussions with the hospital staff and attending physicians. Another trial may require fewer study coordinator hours to record data because the case report form consists of fewer pages.

Institution Charges

Institutions acting as an investigative site for a clinical trial often charge an "overhead," typically a percentage of the total cost of the study. Other institution charges may include a pharmacy department charge for pharmacist participation or study drug storage.

The final study budget should also reflect the cost of anticipated telephone calls, paper supplies, faxing, and other such items. Examples of items to consider are included in the following sample budget-planning chart.

Sample Budget-Planning Chart

Part 1: Patient Charges

List procedures and tests that are outside or in addition to those required for standard care as well as other per patient expenses.

Procedures	# Units Required	Unit Cost	Total Cost
ECG	3	_____	_____
CBC	2	_____	_____
Chest X-ray	1	_____	_____
Pharmacy dispensing	4	_____	_____
Parking passes	4	_____	_____
Total Cost Per Patient		_____	_____

Part 2: Personnel Time

The following example of a chart to determine personnel time is based on a projected enrollment of two patients/week. In this example, the study coordinator would spend approximately 20 hours/week once the start-up phase was complete. Time spent with the monitor during on-site visits would be in addition to the 20 hours per week during the enrollment and maintenance phase of

Personnel	Activity	Estimated Time	Study Phase	Total Hours
Study Coordinator	Review protocol; submit documents to IRB	8 hours	Start-up	8 hours
	Prepare and perform staff inservices	3 hours preparation; 1 hour x 3 presentations	Start-up	6 hours
	Prepare study-specific materials	6 hours	Start-up	6 hours
	Screen and enroll patients	1½ hours / patient	Enrollment and maintenance	3 hours / week
	Conduct follow-up visits	1 hour / patient	Enrollment and maintenance	6 biweekly visits x number of patients
	Complete CRF and other data collection forms	6 hours / patient	Enrollment and maintenance	6 hours x number of patients
	Resolve data queries	1 hour / patient	Maintenance and close-out	1 hour x number of patients
	Communicate with sponsor	1 hour / week	All phases	1 hour per week throughout trial
	Prepare for monitoring visits	2 hours / patient	All phases	2 hours x number of patients
Investigator	Review protocol	2 hours	Start-up	2 hours
	Present protocol at IRB meeting	1 hour	Start-up	1 hour
	Meet with colleagues	2 hours	Start-up	2 hours
	Perform initial screening visit for enrolled patients	1 hour / patient	Enrollment and maintenance	1 hour x number of patients
	Perform follow-up visit	20 minutes / patient visit	Enrollment and maintenance	6 biweekly visits x number of patients
	Communicate with sponsor and staff	1 hour / week	All phases	1 hour per week throughout trial
Support Staff	Call enrolled patients reminder of visits	½ hour / week	Enrollment and maintenance	½ hour / week
	Fax documents; request medical records	½ hour / week	All phases	½ hour / week

the study. The investigator would spend approximately 2 hours/week for study-related activities and support personnel would spend 1 hour/week.

Making the Decision to Be an Investigator/Investigative Site

Finally, after reviewing the protocol and determining the feasibility of implementing this study at your site, ask yourself, "Do I really want to participate in this trial?" The answer to this question may be one of the most important factors in determining the success of a trial. Consider whether this study will be of interest throughout its duration; it will be difficult to maintain enthusiasm if the drug being studied or the question to be answered is of no clinical interest to you. Lack of interest by the investigator, colleagues, and study personnel can result in poor patient enrollment and in reduced trial revenue. It can also affect future participation in clinical trials if sponsors see this work as representative of your site. If there is excitement and motivation to conduct the study, your performance will most likely be enhanced. Enthusiastic participation will lead to a successful study and continued sponsor interest in you and your site.

References

1 Spilker, Bert *Guide to Clinical Trials*, Raven Press, 1991, pg 148

2 Spilker, Bert *Guide to Clinical Trials*, Raven Press, 1991, pg 492

"Never mistake motion for action."

—*Ernest Hemingway*

Study
Activities

9

Each trial has its own infrastructure of individuals and groups responsible for different aspects of the study. Sponsors may assign roles and delegate responsibilities within a clinical trial in numerous ways. These organizational decisions are usually made during the protocol development phase of the trial. Responsibility for aspects such as site monitoring, drug safety, drug or device distribution, site management, and data management may be divided among several groups, including Academic Research Organizations (AROs), Contract Research Organizations (CROs), Site Management Organizations (SMOs), and the sponsor.

The organizational structure will vary from one trial to another based on protocol needs, financial considerations, and logistical issues. While there is no best way to organize the roles and responsibilities within a clinical trial, it is important to be aware of the different groups involved and understand the roles and responsibilities of each. Regardless of the overall organizational structure of the trial, your site's success will depend on a plan that takes into account the uniqueness of your site and the personnel involved in the study.

Sample Organizational Chart

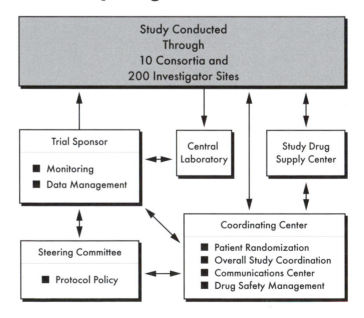

Study Start-up Phase

The start-up phase of a study encompasses the time from when the investigator agrees to participate until the first few patients are enrolled in the study. Collaborate with your study personnel to draw upon their ideas and previous experiences to develop an effective plan for conducting the study. Planning done during this phase will pay off later in the study in areas such as patient recruitment and data collection. The following activities are typically performed during the start-up phase.

Establish the Site Study Team

One of your first responsibilities as an investigator is to establish a site study team, which should include representatives from departments that have protocol-related responsibilities. To determine the study team members, review the protocol carefully and consider the organization of your institution to answer questions such as:

- *Where will patients be identified?*
  When potential patients will be identified in an outpatient clinic or on specific inpatient units, it may be helpful to have personnel from those areas on the study team. Their knowledge and understanding of issues related to their specific areas may help develop a better screening and recruitment plan.

- *Do laboratory samples need to be handled or processed differently from the laboratory routine?*
  When special handling or techniques are required, a laboratory supervisor or designated technician may be identified as a contact person or included on the study team.

■ *Do procedures required for the study need to be performed or documented in a particular manner?*
Trial-related procedures may require non-routine tasks or documentation on specific forms. Personnel from the areas where study procedures will be performed may be able to contribute suggestions to ensure that protocol-designated procedures are followed. For example, if the protocol requires a bicycle exercise test to be performed at a specific pedaling speed or for a specified time period, the technician who routinely sets up the bicycle tests may have some suggestions on how to make sure it is always performed according to protocol.

■ *Can a pharmacist assist with study drug-related issues, drug storage, and drug dispensing?*
The pharmacist may have previous clinical trial experience and be able to provide assistance with study drug issues.

■ *Does the study device need to be stored in a special location?*
A device that requires surgical implantation may need to be stored in a surgical suite; therefore, a designated member of the surgical staff may need to be involved in the planning.

Once you have assembled the site study team, the methods of communication need to be determined, as regular communication throughout the study will be integral to success. During the start-up phase, frequent (weekly) face-to-face meetings may be necessary while developing the study plan. Eventually, the frequency of meetings may decrease as the trial progresses. Sharing study newsletters, enrollment updates, and other communications related to the trial is a good way to keep the study team enthusiastic and informed. Study meetings during start-up might include discussions about enrollment, recruitment issues and strategies, logistical issues such as study-required procedures, and communication from the sponsor. Take minutes of the meetings and distribute them to all team members, and keep a copy in your study file.

Participate in Investigator Meetings

Many sponsors conduct investigator meetings before or just after the first patients are entered into the study. These meetings sometimes serve as a general "initiation visit" (see Chapter 6) with the purpose of educating investigators and study staff about the details of the study. One advantage of reviewing the protocol and required procedures in the setting of an investigator meeting is that questions and discussions raised by individual investigators and study coordinators can benefit the entire group.

Usually, each site's investigator and study coordinator are invited to attend the investigator meeting, which lasts one to two days. Some sponsors also invite other site personnel, such as the site pharmacists, who may have an integral role in the study.

Investigator meetings usually begin with an overview of the study, followed by background information pertinent to the protocol and study treatment, then progressing to a discussion of the specific details of the protocol, including data forms, reporting of serious adverse events, and issues unique to the trial. While some of the sessions are geared toward the study coordinator who often performs many of the trial-related activities, the principal investigator will also benefit from the sessions that reveal the logistical demands of the protocol and provide the opportunity for clinical discussions.

Many investigator meetings are conducted regionally, providing you with the opportunity to meet investigators and coordinators from other participating sites that are located within the same geographic area. These contacts may provide opportunities for additional sources of ideas or information when trying to resolve protocol-related issues in the future. These other sites may also assist or participate when study patients are transferred between institutions.

Develop a Recruitment and Enrollment Plan

Establishing an effective plan for recruiting and enrolling patients will depend greatly upon the patient population, the type of trial, and the individual site. It will be important to provide information about the study to colleagues who may have contact with the target patient population and who may identify potential subjects.

When developing the enrollment plan, consider creating an "enrollment packet" for use when patients are identified. To determine the forms that should be included in the packet, review the steps of the screening and enrollment process for the study. Documents and forms to consider placing in the enrollment packet include:

- Screening/enrollment forms

- Consent form

- Medical record release forms

- Patient contact information sheets

- Worksheets created for study-related procedures

- Physician orders for study-related procedures and tests

Place the packets in the locations where patients will be screened and enrolled.

In acute trials where enrollment must occur within a narrow time frame, a number of tools have proven helpful in quickly screening and identifying patients. One of these tools is a pocket reference card for physicians and nurses that outlines eligibility criteria and provides a quick review of protocol-required procedures. Posters that provide the same information may be placed in a visible location in areas where staff will be identifying patients. When randomization is performed by calling a specified telephone number, stickers with the randomization telephone number may be attached to the telephones at various locations.

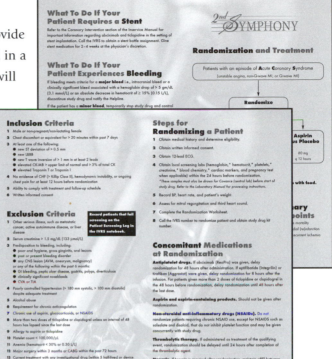

For non-acute trials or outpatient studies, additional methods for recruiting patients might include letters to colleagues about the study and radio or newspaper advertisements for potential patients. Advertisements should be simple and limited to information a subject needs to know to determine eligibility and interest, and must be reviewed and approved by the institutional review board before use.

The FDA views recruitment of subjects as an extension of the informed consent process and requires advertisements to include the following elements:

1 name and address of the investigator and research facility conducting the study;

2 purpose of research and summary of the eligibility criteria for study enrollment;

3 condensed description of the benefits enrolled subjects receive;

4 contact name and number for additional information.

Avoid the following in advertisements:

1 claims that the drug or device is safe or effective for the indication under investigation;

2 use of the terms "new treatment," "new medication," or "new drugs" without explaining that the test article is investigational (21 CFR § 312.7a);

3 emphasis on financial rewards for study participation such as money paid to the subject or free medical treatment. This may be viewed as coercive to financially-constrained patients.

Sample Advertisement

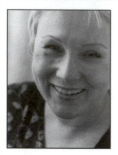

Do you take insulin for your Diabetes?

Have you taken insulin for more than 1 year?

Do you take a single dose of insulin in the morning?

Do you test your blood sugar daily?

If you are between 40 and 80 years of age and meet study criteria, you may be eligible to participate in a research study of an investigational medication at your local hospital. A new type of insulin is being evaluated for the treatment of insulin-dependent diabetes. Study medication and physical assessments will be provided free of charge for this 90-day study. For more information call *<local contact name>* at *<phone number and hospital name>*.

Competing Trials at Your Site

One challenge to study recruitment is other trials at your site competing for the same patient population. When this occurs, enrolling sufficient patients in your trial may be difficult. There is also a chance that selection bias can be introduced into one or both studies, since competing trials may promote an unconscious (or conscious!) decision about which protocol better suits an individual patient. Therefore, if competing trials do exist at your site, make efforts to ensure that enrollment in both trials is based on objective criteria.

Two such methods are:

1 limiting enrollment in one trial to even days and to the second trial on odd days, and

2 alternating enrollment in trials as eligible patients are identified.

These options are not perfect, and obviously reduce potential enrollment in both trials, but may be necessary if your site is involved in competing trials.

Conduct Educational Inservices for Site Personnel

Once the enrollment plan has been established, it will be easier to identify site personnel who need to be aware of the study procedures and details. If your study involves acutely ill or hospitalized patients, patient care staff on all shifts will need to be informed about the study, as will clinic staff when outpatient studies are performed. Topics to review during the inservice should include the purpose of the study, the patient population, required procedures, and data documentation. The importance of protocol adherence and the collection of necessary data should be stressed to all personnel.

To inform your colleagues about the study, consider scheduling a presentation at grand rounds or similar meetings. Sponsors will often provide slides that can be used at these presentations. Give colleagues and personnel working with the target population a written summary of the study that provides information on how to contact the investigator and study coordinator.

You may want to develop study materials in addition to those supplied by the sponsor. A review of the patient data forms should identify data that are not routinely collected or documented at your site. These might include laboratory samples required at atypical times, or physical assessment requirements different from the routine of the site clinicians.

Sample Worksheet

For some studies, creating simple reminders or worksheets will help staff obtain the required data without significantly increasing their workload. Worksheets can serve as a reminder to ensure that protocol-designated procedures are performed and completed appropriately, especially important when study procedures fall outside the routine. A telephone or pager number of the person to be contacted when questions arise outside of work hours should be available to site personnel.

Randomize and Enroll Patients

Patient enrollment can begin once the site staff has been oriented to the study. A consent form signed by the patient must be obtained before initiating any protocol-required procedures, and a copy must be provided to the patient (refer to Chapter 4 for additional details on the informed consent process).

TIP: It may be helpful to have the patient sign a *release of medical information form* at the time of enrollment. This will be useful if the patient is later transferred to another institution and study-related data need to be obtained from the other institution.

Patient contact information should also be collected as soon as possible after enrollment to provide the study coordinator with telephone numbers to call when scheduling follow-up visits.

Once the first few patients have been enrolled, review the enrollment process to identify the components that worked well and those that were not as successful. Adjustments to the enrollment process or enrollment packet should be made as early as possible so that a revised plan is in place to enroll subsequent patients.

Study Maintenance Phase

After processes have been established and the first few patients have been enrolled, you gradually move into what can be referred to as the maintenance phase of the study. During this phase, activities include the completion of data collection forms as well as continued screening and enrollment of patients. You will need to address trial-related concerns as they arise and maintain enthusiasm for the study.

Complete Data Forms

Timely completion and submission of the patient data forms is an important activity during the maintenance phase. In some studies, an interim analysis is performed on data at pre-determined timepoints; major decisions, such as whether the trial should be modified or continued as-is, are based on the data reviewed in this analysis. The sponsor or data center usually provides instructions on how and when forms should be completed and submitted.

From a practical point of view, it is best to record the data on the forms as they become available. As you complete data forms for the first few patients, you will be able to identify areas where data are not being recorded in your source documents. With this information, you can take corrective action to ensure the data are available for future patients. Actions might include developing a worksheet to remind patient-care providers when vital signs need to be evaluated, or requesting that staff record data in the patient medical record. Chapter 12 discusses the data collection process in greater detail.

Report Serious Adverse Events

The protocol or other study documents will outline serious adverse events that may require expedited reporting in the study. Events that require expedited reporting may vary widely from one trial to the next, so familiarize yourself with the requirements and event definitions for the specific trial. This is an important safety issue for all patients enrolled in the study and requires vigilance on the part of participating investigators. Detailed information regarding adverse events is found in Chapter 5.

Conduct Patient Follow-up Visits

Studies that involve multiple follow-up visits over a long period of time offer a unique set of challenges to the investigative site. Visits must be planned and tests or procedures needed at the time of the follow-up visit must be coordinated and scheduled. Be aware of the requirements for each visit so that appropriate time is allotted for procedures to be performed. The use of worksheets, checklists, and study calendars will help in planning to ensure protocol adherence. To facilitate the planning of follow-up visits consider the following suggestions:

■ Establish a location and times when the investigator and study coordinator are both available.

- Confirm that protocol-required procedures, such as blood drawing or exercise testing, can be performed during the time allotted for the scheduled visit.

- Provide the patient with an appointment card or a study calendar with scheduled appointments.

- Call or send a reminder card to patients before each appointment.

- Establish a system for tracking each patient's scheduled appointments, completed appointments, and missed or cancelled appointments.

- Contact the patient by telephone when there is a long span between visits. Ask if the patient has any trial-related questions, and take the opportunity to reinforce the importance of participation in the study.

Visit Tracking Log

FEH's
For our Examples: a Hypothetical Study

- Record scheduled date in pencil; record in ink when visit has been completed.
- Contact patient a week before scheduled visit as a reminder.
- Schedule ECG and blood samples for morning of visit.

Enrollment Visit 1 Week 0	Pt. Initials	Study Number	Randomization Visit 2 Week 1	Visit 3 Week 2	Visit 4 Week 4	Visit 5 Week 6	Visit 6 Week 8	Study Completion Visit 7 Week 12
08/JAN/2001	XYZ	001	15/JAN/2001	22/JAN/2001	05/FEB/2001	19/FEB/2001	05/MAR/2001	
17/JAN/2001	ABC	002	24/JAN/2001	31/JAN/2001	14/FEB/2001	28/FEB/2001		
02/FEB/2001	CDE	003	09/FEB/2001	16/FEB/2001	23/FEB/2001			
21/FEB/2001	PDQ	004	28/FEB/2001	07/MAR/2001				

Ensure Patient Compliance

Just as keeping site study team members informed is critical to the success of the study, keeping enrolled patients informed about the trial is also vital. Sending visit reminders, telephoning patients between visits, or providing a patient newsletter are ways to maintain patient interest in a study. Reminding patients of what to expect during each visit (time commitment, blood draws, special tests, etc.) will help foster cooperation and minimize frustration. If necessary, establish special clinic hours (during the lunch hour, before or after work) to maximize patient compliance. Establishing a positive and helpful relationship with study participants will be invaluable in

Sample Patient Contact Information Sheet

gaining full cooperation and ensuring that patients complete their full course of study therapy.

To facilitate patient retention:

■ explain study and length of commitment thoroughly at time of enrollment;

■ involve the patient's family in discussions;

■ discuss visit frequency and approximate time commitment for study;

■ discuss and solve transportation issues (provide parking vouchers, explore public transportation).

There may be times when you will be unable to locate patients enrolled in the study when follow-up is required. Use the patient contact information obtained at the time of enrollment to identify a friend or relative not living with the patient or the physician responsible for ongoing care. One of these individuals may know the patient's whereabouts.

■ Call at various times during the day, at home or work, over the course of several weeks.

■ Contact the primary or referring physician.

■ Contact the individual not living with the patient listed on the patient contact information sheet.

FEHs
For our Examples: a Hypothetical Study

Protocol-Study #: _____ - _____   **Visit 1**   Patient's Initials: ___ ___ ___   Allocation #: __ __ __ __ __
                 protocol number site number   first middle last

Contacts

Patient Contact Information (please print)

Patient Identification

Patient name: _____ / _____ / _____
                        Last   First   Middle

Social security number: _____
Resident identification number: _____   Medical record number: _____
Primary home address: _____
                      _____
                      _____

Primary home phone number: _____   → Best time to call: _____ ☐ AM ☐ PM
Business phone number: _____ → Best time to call: ☐ AM ☐ PM
E-mail address: _____
Spouse or significant other: _____ / _____ / _____
                             Last   First   Middle
Spouse/significant other business name: _____
Spouse/significant other business phone number: _____
E-mail address: _____

Secondary Residence (vacation home, etc.)
Mailing address: _____
                 _____

Phone number: _____   → Best time to call: _____ ☐ AM ☐ PM

Alternative Contacts *(please list two relatives, friends or neighbors not living with patient)*

1 Name: _____ / _____ / _____
          Last   First   Middle
Relationship to patient: _____
Mailing address: _____
                 _____

Phone number: _____   → Best time to call: _____ ☐ AM ☐ PM
E-mail address: _____

2 Name: _____ / _____ / _____
          Last   First   Middle
Relationship to patient: _____
Mailing address: _____
                 _____

Phone number: _____   → Best time to call: _____ ☐ AM ☐ PM
E-mail address: _____

Local/Referring Physician or Primary Care Physician/General Practitioner

Name: _____ / _____ / _____
       Last   First   Middle
Mailing address: _____
                 _____

Physician's office phone number: _____   Office fax number: _____

Contains confidential patient information. Do NOT fax or send this page with patient's case report form.

18 July 2000   **FEHs** Contacts

- Review hospital medical record/emergency contact/next-of-kin information.

- Call the local telephone company directory information.

- Send a certified letter to the patient and/or the individual not living with the patient.

Unblind Study Treatment Only When Required

The underlying philosophy for unblinding study treatment is that it should occur only when knowledge of the treatment code will influence decisions about patient care. More often, the unblinding of study treatment is not necessary, and the appropriate decision for patient management is to discontinue the study drug, reduce the dose, or temporarily stop study drug as indicated in the protocol. Unblinding study treatment rarely adds further information that affects patient care.

Studies that are blinded to both the investigator and the patient must provide a mechanism to unblind study medication in the case of a patient emergency when it is essential to know which study treatment the patient received. There are a variety of ways that unblinding can occur. Some of these methods are: 1) calling a specific number with 24-hour availability, 2) envelopes containing the patient treatment information that may be kept in a secured location at the site, and 3) scratch-off or wipe-off labels on the study drug containers. Instructions about the appropriate unblinding procedure for the study will be provided in the protocol, by the sponsor, or by the designated study pharmacy.

9. Study Activities

Obtain Answers to Urgent Clinical Questions

Many studies have a "helpline" telephone number where clinicians are on call 24 hours a day to assist in making clinical decisions regarding potential patient eligibility or managing an urgent clinical problem for a patient enrolled in the study. Typically, questions posed to the helpline should be urgent and about real patients, not hypothetical situations. Additional contact numbers are generally provided for non-urgent study-related questions, such as those regarding the completion of data forms.

Continue Communication

During this phase of the study you will be in contact with the monitor and/or site management team designated by the sponsor. Regular communication serves to update the site as to the progress of the overall study, to relay helpful information, and to check the status of data forms. Some sponsors may provide newsletters or faxes to provide new information about the study and provide helpful hints to all sites. You may choose to share this information with appropriate personnel at your site as a way of maintaining their enthusiasm for the study.

Maintain Study File

Throughout the course of the study, the site study file needs to be kept up-to-date. Communications, reports, and other information pertinent to the study should be filed on an ongoing basis throughout the study. Refer to Chapter 10 for further information on study documents.

Study Completion and Close-out Phase

Eventually, patient recruitment will be complete and the sponsor will begin the process of closing out the trial at participating sites. Many trial-related activities continue after recruitment has been completed, including the continued recording and submission of patient data. Follow-up visits often must be scheduled after completion of enrollment, and patient care issues may still surface. The study close-out process may be performed during an on-site monitoring visit, or may take place via telephone, computer, or fax, with the use of checklists to ensure that all activities have been completed.

Ongoing communication with the sponsor, the monitor, and the site study team is an important aspect during the close-out phase. Provide feedback to the site personnel and study staff who participated in the study. When study results become known, share this information with the staff at your site, including nursing and pharmacy personnel, laboratory staff, and others who worked with study patients and performed study procedures. This serves both to provide the trial results to the many personnel who participated in the study as well as to acknowledge their contributions.

What Happens at Close-out?

- Completion of all case report forms and resolution of data queries

- Destruction or return of study materials and drug/device as directed by the sponsor

- A review of the site study file to confirm completeness

- Submission of the final report to the IRB and the sponsor

- Long-term storage of study records and study file

"The purpose of medicine is to prevent significant disease, to decrease pain and to postpone death when it is meaningful to do so. Technology has to support these goals—if not, it may even be counterproductive."

—*Dr. Joel J. Nobel*, **"On the Development and Maintenance of High-technology Medical Systems"**

Study Documents

To ensure accountability by investigators and institutional review boards, the FDA requires specific documentation from all investigators each time they participate in a clinical trial conducted under an Investigational New Drug (IND) application or an Investigational Device Exemption (IDE). In addition to the documentation required by the FDA, there may be other forms and documents requested by sponsors to meet internal standards and requirements, as well as additional regulatory requirements for federally funded trials. Keep all trial-related documents in your study file, with the exception of the contractual agreement (the financial contract that outlines site payments from the sponsor), which should be filed separately. Trial-related documents must be available for review by the sponsor and FDA throughout and following the study.

The following sections describe documents used in investigational drug trials conducted under an IND. The documents required for trials of devices studied under an IDE (Investigational Device Exemption) application, and biological products conducted under a PLA (Product License Application), as well as those required for post-marketing studies will be different from the documents listed below. For example, one of the differences between IND and IDE study documents is that the Form FDA 1572 (Statement of Investigator) is required only for IND (drug) studies, not for device studies. Refer to 21 CFR § 812 for investigational device exemption requirements and to 21 CFR § 600–680 for biologic product requirements.

Documents Required at Study Start-up

Many factors, including the sponsor and the type of trial, determine the order in which your site receives and completes documents and may vary from one trial to another. When approached about participating in a clinical trial as a principal investigator, you may be required to sign a confidentiality agreement before being given a copy of the protocol to review. This agreement between the investigator and the sponsor requires the investigator to keep the contents of the protocol confidential and any other proprietary information regarding the study. Once the confidentiality agreement has been signed, you will receive a protocol to review. If you subsequently agree to be an investigator in the trial, additional documents will be sent. Some of these are required by regulatory requirements, while others may be sponsor-required forms.

In an investigational drug trial, the FDA requires that the sponsor obtain from each investigator:

1 The investigator's Curriculum Vitae (CV) and the completed Form FDA 1572 signed by the investigator

2 Evidence of IRB approval for both the protocol and the consent form

3 Financial disclosure information

The sponsor may require these additional items:

1 A photocopy of the IRB-approved consent form

2 Letter of agreement (also called investigator agreement or protocol signature page)

3 Financial contract (also called contractual agreement)

4 Laboratory certification form and laboratory normal ranges form

5 Site demographics form

6 Medical licensure form

7 Study personnel résumés and training records

Form FDA 1572 and Curriculum Vitae

The Form FDA 1572 must be completed and signed by each principal investigator participating in a clinical trial being conducted under an IND. This form is a contract between the investigator and the FDA; by signing it, you agree to adhere to the regulations governing clinical research and conduct the study according to the protocol. The original Form FDA 1572 is collected by the sponsor and is ultimately submitted to the FDA by the sponsor. Correction fluid may not be used on the Form FDA 1572.

IRB Approval

The first step in initiating a study at your site is submitting the protocol, investigator's brochure, and consent form to the Investigational Review Board (IRB) for approval. If the sponsor supplies a sample consent form, fill in the consent form with local names and contact information before submitting it to the IRB. Patient recruitment materials and advertisements must be submitted and approved by the IRB before use. The IRB will review the information and may ask questions about the study, request additional information, or ask for revisions to be made to the consent form, advertisements, or other materials before giving approval.

IRB Approval Letter

When the IRB approves a study, the IRB must provide the investigator with a letter documenting approval to conduct the study at the site. The IRB letter must specifically state the name and date of the protocol, and the protocol version number. Written IRB approval of advertisements must also be documented. The IRB usually includes other specific instructions in the approval letter, such as the time period of approval and the frequency of expected reporting to the IRB. Approval for the protocol, the consent form, and other applicable documents such as advertisements and assent forms are often included in one letter; however, they may be stated in separate letters, and consent form approval may be stamped and dated on a blank copy of the consent form. Submit a copy of the IRB approval letter to the sponsor, and keep the original in the site study file.

May 12, 2000

Dear Dr. Candoit,

The study protocol known as FEHS (For our Example: a Hypothetical Study) Protocol # 24687-CH dated March 10, 2000, and the study consent form Version 1 dated March 30, 2000, have been approved by the Institutional Review Board of Anytown Hospital on May 8, 2000.

As a reminder, no protocol changes may be implemented without first obtaining written IRB approval. Unanticipated problems and serious adverse events must be promptly reported to the IRB. The protocol will be due for review 12 months from the date of approval.

Sincerely,

Dr. Ina Approve
Chairperson, Institutional Review Board

At right is an example of an IRB letter indicating study approval. The components mentioned above must be included in the letter.

IRB approval letters are reviewed during on-site monitoring visits and may also be reviewed by the FDA during site inspections as part of the site regulatory files.

TIP: Make sure your approval letter includes a protocol date in the letter and written approval for the consent form.

155

IRB Membership Documentation

The site study file should also include a list of the IRB members. In some cases, IRBs do not allow the members' names to be given out, and will instead supply a statement that the IRB meets and complies with all the regulations regarding IRBs. When this is the case, submit the statement to the sponsor and keep a copy in the study file.

If the investigator or study coordinator is a voting member of the IRB, documentation that he or she was not involved in the voting for IRB approval for the designated study should be recorded and filed.

Financial Disclosure Information

Regulations effective as of February 1999 require the sponsor to collect financial disclosure information from each investigator participating in a clinical study of drugs, biologics, and devices. For investigational drug studies, this information must be collected from each investigator listed in sections 1 and 6 of the Form FDA 1572. The information about financial interest in the sponsor or study to be disclosed applies to the investigators, their spouses, and their dependents. Refer to Chapter 3 for additional information about financial disclosure.

Consent Form

The consent form—including assent forms for children, the "short form" version of a consent form, and the written summary that corresponds to the short form—should be submitted to the IRB for approval along with the protocol. Approval of the consent form may be stated in the IRB letter approving the protocol, or the consent form itself may be stamped "Approved" and dated and initialed by the IRB chairperson. Verification that the consent form was approved by the IRB should be forwarded to the sponsor.

Check with your site's medical records department to ensure that the consent form meets hospital/institution archiving specifications. Patient-signed consent forms that are kept in the patient's hospital record are sometimes discarded by the medical records department if not printed on hospital letterhead or approved by the institution's internal forms committee. Keep either the original signed consent form or a copy of the original in the site study file in addition to a consent form kept in the patient's hospital record or clinic chart.

Letter of Agreement

Just as the Form FDA 1572 is a contract between the investigator and the FDA in an investigational drug study, the letter of agreement is a contract between the investigator and the study sponsor. The details of the contract are sometimes spelled out in an actual "letter of agreement" or may be a copy of the "signature page" of the protocol requiring signatures from both a sponsor representative and the investigator. By signing the protocol signature page or a letter of agreement, you are promising the sponsor that you will conduct the study according to the design of the protocol and in accordance with the regulations governing clinical research.

Financial Contract

The financial contract between the investigator and the sponsor identifies when and how much the site will be paid for trial-related activities. Amounts paid to sites for study participation may vary based on the actual charges and costs at different institutions and locations. The contract should specify the frequency and timing of payments, the milestones that a site must reach to generate a payment, and when final payment will be made. The financial contract is usually kept separate from the study file.

Laboratory Certification and Normal Ranges Form

When laboratory samples are processed at the institution or a local laboratory and results recorded on the data collection forms, the sponsor may require a copy of the certification indicating that the laboratory meets the current standards for handling and processing samples. Laboratory certification is required under the CLIA (Clinical Laboratory Improvement Act of 1988) and is usually issued by the College of American Pathologists (CAP). When the sponsor requires certification, copies of the certificates should be obtained from all laboratories that will be processing samples included as part of the patient data. Certification is performed by the state (and sometimes the city) where the laboratories are located, and usually covers a 2- to 3-year period. Be sure to obtain a copy of the renewal letter or certificate if the laboratory certification expires during the study.

Sample Lab Normals Form

In some trials, a laboratory normal ranges form must be completed, providing normal ranges for the laboratory results recorded on the patient data collection forms. This provides a reference for comparing the reported patient values. If these ranges change during the trial due to new laboratory equipment or other reasons, updated ranges should be collected and provided to the sponsor, with a copy kept in your site study file.

Site Demographics Form

Also called a site information sheet, this form provides the sponsor with the names, telephone numbers, and addresses of trial-related personnel, and other general information about your site. This information identifies where and to whom correspondence, study drug, and study materials should be shipped. It is important to update this form when names, numbers, and/or addresses change during a study.

Medical Licensure Form

Some sponsors require the current medical license numbers for the investigator and sub-investigators. Sponsors may request a photocopy of the investigator's medical license or may provide a medical licensure form on which to record this information.

Study Personnel Résumés and Training Records

Some sponsors will request copies of the résumés and training records of study personnel at the site. The résumés document the qualifications of the study coordinator and others to whom you have delegated study responsibilities, while training records indicate specific education and training

10. Study Documents

159

pertinent to clinical research and even more specifically to the trial. Documentation of attendees at inservices conducted by the investigator and study coordinator identifies study-specific training provided to site personnel.

Documents Required While the Study is in Progress

As a trial progresses, you may be required to submit and file additional documents. These will depend on issues that arise during the study and may include the following:

Protocol Amendments

If changes are made to the approved protocol, an amendment must be submitted to the IRB and approval obtained before the protocol changes can be implemented. Changes that require a protocol amendment can be found in 21 CFR § 312.30.

Expedited Review

While every amendment requires IRB approval, not every amendment must be reviewed by the entire IRB committee for approval. The FDA has created a list of research categories that may be reviewed by the IRB through an *expedited review* procedure. This list is published in the Federal Register and updated as needed.

An IRB may use the *expedited review* process to review either or both of the following:

Protocol Changes Requiring an Amendment:

- an increase in the study drug dose or duration,

- a significant change in the study design (such as adding or dropping a control group), or

- the addition of a test or procedure even when its intent is to reduce the risk of or improve the monitoring for an adverse event (for example, testing serum creatinine at additional timepoints if kidney function needs to be closely observed).[1]

1 Some or all of the research can be found on the published list of research categories, and the research is found to involve no more than minimal risk.

2 There are minor changes to a research study approved within the previous 12 months.[2]

Under an expedited review procedure, the IRB chairperson or one or more experienced reviewers designated by the chairperson may perform the review. The reviewers may exercise all of the authorities of the IRB except to disapprove the study, which can only occur in accordance with a non-expedited review. The IRB must have in place a system to notify the full committee of the approval when expedited review is implemented. The IRB chairman also has the right to request a full IRB review of any protocol amendment.

Once IRB approval for an amendment is obtained, a copy of the amendment and the approval letter must be kept in your study file and a copy of the IRB approval letter forwarded to the sponsor.

Revised Consent Forms

If the original approved consent form is revised for any reason during the trial (for example, due to a safety issue or a protocol change), the revised consent form must be approved by the IRB. This revised consent form must be used to obtain consent from all study subjects enrolled after IRB approval has been received. Some protocol and consent form revisions may affect subjects currently enrolled in the study, such as when additional blood tests are required, the visit schedule is changed, or study drug dosing is altered. When this occurs, all previously enrolled subjects must be informed of the changes and sign the revised IRB-approved consent form, indicating willingness to continue participation in the study. A copy of the revised consent form and all previously approved versions must be kept in the study file. Be sure that the current version of the consent form is easily identifiable by a date and version number located on each page.

Keep a copy of the signed consent form for all enrolled subjects in your site study file. Depending on the type of trial and monitoring that will be performed, the sponsor may recommend that you keep signed consent forms in a central location in the study file or that each consent form be kept with the individual patient case report form. Some institutions require the original consent form to be filed in the patient's medical record, while others recommend keeping the original in the site study file with a photocopy in the medical record. Be sure to determine your institution's policy in order to comply with local requirements.

Updated Form FDA 1572

Changes that require a new Form FDA 1572 to be completed include:

1 Changes in the investigator name or address

2 Changes in the IRB address

3 The addition of sub-investigators, local laboratories, or locations where patient visits will be conducted

When Form FDA 1572 information is updated, a new form must be completed in entirety, signed and dated, and submitted to the sponsor. A copy of the new Form FDA 1572 should be kept in your site study file with a copy of the initial Form FDA 1572. Note that in addition to revising the Form FDA 1572, full IRB review must also occur when the principal investigator changes.

IRB Correspondence

In addition to the items originally submitted to the IRB, all additional communication with the IRB should be kept in your study file. This includes:

- *Trial Progress Reports*—Reports provided to the IRB by the investigator summarizing trial progress to date. The frequency of these reports is determined by the individual IRB, and may be based on the degree of risk involved with the study.

- *Annual IRB Renewals*—Documents submitted by the investigator to obtain continued approval to conduct the study. The regulations require each protocol to be renewed by the IRB at least annually; some IRBs request more frequent review. Submit the IRB letter documenting continued study approval to the sponsor.

- *IND Safety Reports*—Reports generated by the sponsor and sent to all site investigators when a safety issue occurs. A copy of IND Safety Reports should be forwarded to your IRB; documentation of IRB notification should be kept in your study file with a copy of the IND Safety Report.

Patient Recruitment Advertisements

New advertisements and changes to previously approved recruitment materials must be approved by the IRB. Keep copies of all advertisements (such as flyers, newspaper ads, and text for radio announcements) in the study file with documentation of IRB approval. See Chapter 9 for specific information about advertisements.

Sample Screening Log

Screening Log

Sponsors may require each site to complete a screening log to list all subjects who were screened for study enrollment, including those who were not enrolled. The log should be updated continually throughout the trial identifying the reasons that potential subjects are not enrolled.

Patient Master Log

A Master Log may be provided as a mechanism to record all subjects enrolled in the study. The log can function as a tool to record subject contact information, providing the necessary information when subjects must be contacted at any time during or after the study. In addition to contacting subjects to schedule outpatient visits and follow-up, subjects may need to be contacted if study safety concerns arise, or if new information that might affect a subject's willingness to continue participation becomes available.

Sample Patient Master Log

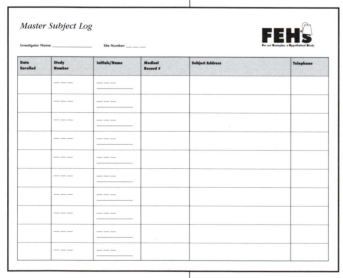

Drug Accountability Forms

Documentation of the receipt and dispensing of study supplies must be updated throughout the study. Usually the sponsor provides drug accountability, dispensing, and invoicing forms. If these are not supplied, your institution's pharmacy forms may be used as long as the appropriate information is documented. Refer to Chapter 11 for additional information about study drug and accountability forms.

Reportable Adverse Event Forms

In each study, sponsors designate certain adverse experiences as events that must be reported in an expedited manner. Examples of events that might require expedited reporting include death, stroke, thrombocytopenia, and anaphylactic shock; these events will vary based on trial design and phase. Report forms are typically completed and faxed to the sponsor within 24 hours of the investigator learning of the event. This early reporting system allows the sponsor to obtain information in a timely manner consistent with the regulatory requirements, rather than at a much later date when data forms are submitted.

Keep copies of all completed expedited adverse event reports submitted to the sponsor in your study file. Follow-up adverse event information that is reported to the sponsor should be filed, as well as documentation of IRB notification when applicable. Chapter 5 contains additional information about adverse events and reporting requirements.

Patient Data Forms and Query Forms

Throughout the study, patient data forms, such as case report forms, follow-up forms, and patient questionnaires must be completed and submitted to the sponsor or data center. Copies of all initial data forms and subsequent changes to the data must be kept at the site. Changes to the data after the data forms have been submitted may be initiated by site study personnel or by data management personnel, when incorrect data, missing data, or data that are outside the expected range of responses are identified.

When the data center sends query forms listing the data in question, the site study personnel must review the data identified, and either confirm the original data or make corrections. Specific instructions for returning the query forms to the data center (usually by fax or mail) will be provided. Instructions for correcting data errors that are identified by the site should also be provided. The data center should also provide specific instructions on whether corrections should be made only on the query forms or directly on the site's copy of the case report form. Carefully follow the instructions provided so that the data forms at the site match those at the sponsor and data center.

Sample Site Signature Log

FEHs				
For our Example: a Hypothetical Study		Site Name: _____		Site Number: __ __
Title *(PI, Coordinator, Pharmacist, etc.)*	**Role on FEHs**	**Printed Name**	**Signature**	**Initials**

Site Signature Log

At the end of the study, mail the top page to FEHs Coordination Team
04/OCT/2000

Signature Log

The signature log is a form used to record the signature and initials of all individuals who record data on the patient data forms or query forms during the trial. Signature lists may also be used to document staff authority to perform study procedures, as delegated by the investigator.

Monitoring Log

Monitors—the individuals who are designated to perform on-site visits and oversee the progress of the trial at the site—sign this log when conducting an on-site visit (see

Chapter 6). The log typically provides a place to document the date and type of visit, and the name of the person conducting the visit.

Written Communication and Correspondence

All communication about the study, including newsletters and faxes sent as updates during the course of the trial, should be kept in the study file. Include all reports from monitoring visits and other communication with the sponsor. Written documentation of telephone communication, including discussions with "helpline" personnel, monitors, the sponsor, and the data center, should be kept and filed.

Documents Required at Study Close-out

A number of documents will be required at the end of the study. Depending on the trial, the monitor may collect documents at the final on-site monitoring visit, or the site may be asked to submit final documents to the sponsor by mail, fax, or courier.

Outstanding Data Forms and Query Forms

Inconsistencies or errors on the data collection forms can be identified long after the study is completed. These issues must be resolved so that accurate and complete data are submitted to the FDA.

Final Reports

The IRB and the sponsor both require the site to submit a final report. The format and specific content of the IRB final report may be determined by the IRB, but generally includes the date the study is completed, the number of patients enrolled, and the types and severity of any adverse events including serious, unexpected, or life-threatening events. The report should include a comment that all patients have completed study-related treatment or have completed participation in the study.

The sponsor may accept a copy of the report to the IRB as their final report, or may require a format different from that of the IRB. The regulations require that the final report be submitted within a "timely manner" for investigational drug trials, and within three months of study completion for device trials.

Sample Final Report

February 17, 2001

IRB Chairperson
Medical Center
Anytown, USA

Re: IRB # 2345-01 A Randomized, Double-Blind, Multicenter, Placebo-Controlled Study of Drug XX on Hemodynamics In Patients With Class IV Heart Failure

Dear IRB Chairperson:

This letter serves as notification of the closure of enrollment and the completion of patient follow-up at our institution in the study noted above. Enrollment ended February 2, 2001, with a total of 135 patients. The sponsor estimates that 30 day follow-up will be completed at all remaining sites by the end of March, 2001. Ten patients were consented and enrolled in this study at our institution. Of these ten patients, there were five Caucasian males, two Native American males, two African American males, and one African American female. None of the patients withdrew prematurely.

During the course of this study, the Institutional Review Board was notified of two sponsor-reported serious adverse events in a letter dated November 6, 2000. In addition to these two events, one serious adverse event occurred at our institution. The IRB was notified December 1, 2000, regarding the subject RDU (#003) who developed sepsis, with blood and urine cultures positive for E.Coli. This event was believed unlikely to be related to study medication. The patient recovered and was discharged home with no sequelae.

There was one amendment to the original protocol, dated April 08, 2000, that added a dyspnea scale to be performed 8 hours after study drug administration. IRB approval was received April 30, 2000.

There are no preliminary results from the trial at this time. No sponsor audits or FDA inspections were performed during this study. We will notify the IRB at the time of study completion nationwide, probably sometime in April, 2001.

Please contact me if you have any questions. Your signature below indicates receipt of this letter; please forward a copy to me for our study files. Thank you for your attention to these matters.

_____   _____
Principal Investigator   Chairman, Institutional Review Board

Drug Accountability Records

The sponsor determines if unused or damaged study drug and study articles should be shipped to a designated location at the end of the study or destroyed at the site. If destroyed on-site, an institutional SOP (Standard Operating Procedure) for the destruction of clinical test materials is needed. Instructions will be provided to document the final disposition of all supplies on the appropriate accountability forms.

Maintaining a Study File

The forms and documents listed above should all be included in your site study file. This file should be created at the beginning of the study and updated as the study progresses. Keep all versions of each document in the file; for example, both the original IRB-approved consent form and a revised IRB-approved consent form should be kept.

Record Retention

The site study file and patient data forms must be kept for at least two years following the approval of a New Drug Application (NDA). If the sponsor decides not to file an NDA, the storage period requirement is two years after the sponsor notifies the FDA that the study has been discontinued. Some sponsors require longer record retention—up to 15 years for some international trials! This ensures that the data are available for review by the sponsor or FDA if needed. Check with the sponsor to ensure record retention for the appropriate period of time.

If you relocate after study enrollment is complete, the study file and trial records may be transferred to another individual at the same institution who is willing to accept responsibility for maintaining the records for the required time period. The sponsor must be notified in writing of the name and address of the individual assuming responsibility. If no one at the site is willing or able to accept responsibility for the documents, you must take the documents to your new location and notify the sponsor of the new address. If this is not an option, discuss other alternatives for record retention with the sponsor. Be certain to contact the sponsor before any study records are destroyed.

Principal Investigator Status Change

If you relocate during the study but name a replacement investigator, you must notify the IRB to obtain a full IRB committee review, and submit a new Form FDA 1572 to the sponsor listing the new investigator. If a replacement investigator cannot be identified, the sponsor must be notified and the study discontinued at that site. The sponsor will provide instructions on how to close out the study.

Sample Study File Organization

The following is an example of the organization of a site study file. The monitor will review this file during on-site visits.

 Protocol and Amendments

- Copy of each protocol version
- Protocol amendments
- Signed investigator agreement/protocol signature page

 Signed Form FDA 1572

- Curriculum vitae of principal investigator
- Updated Form FDA 1572

 Investigator's Brochure (all versions) /Investigational Drug Brochure

Institutional Review Board (IRB)

- IRB membership list including their affiliations and terms of office or letter stating the IRB meets all requirements

- Initial submission letter and protocol documents requesting approval

- IRB letter stating approval of protocol and consent form

- Letters and revised documents (protocol amendments and revised consent forms) submitted for approval

- IRB letter stating approval of protocol amendments and revised consent forms

- Copies of approved subject recruitment advertisements

- IND Safety Reports and associated letters to IRB from PI

- Reports to IRB about progress of study (at IRB specified timepoints)

- Final reports to IRB and sponsor

Consent Form

- Blank copy of all approved versions of the consent form

- Copies of signed consent forms for all enrolled patients

Screening Log/Master Log

Laboratory Certification and Laboratory Normal Ranges Form

Drug accountability

- Shipping invoice/receipt of study drug records

- Inventory log

- Dispensing log

- Records of disposition and/or return of unused or damaged study drug

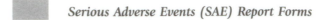 *Serious Adverse Events (SAE) Report Forms*

■ Blank copy of SAE report form

■ Copies of all completed SAE report forms for enrolled patients

Protocol Signature Page

Monitoring Log

General Correspondence

■ Letters

■ Memorandums

■ Written documentation of telephone conversations

■ Facsimiles

■ Electronic communication between the site and the monitor, sponsor, and other trial related groups

References

1 21CFR § 312.3 and 21 CFR 812.3(o)

2 21CFR § 56.110

"A corrected Anti-Epileptic Water of Languis. Take shavings of man's scull, mistletoe of the oak, roots of piony, and white dittany, of each two ounces; fresh flowers of lilly convally, two handfuls; of lavender, rosemary, and tilet, of each three handfuls; cinnamon, six drams; nutmeg, half an ounce; cloves, mace, and cubebs, of each two drams; being all bruised, put them into a matras close stopp'd, in eight pints of malmsey; let them macerate for a week over a very gentle fire; then distill them on a moderate sand-bath, and keep the water for use."

—*From Moses Charras's* Royal Pharmacopoeia. *Translated in English. London 1678*

Study Drug Management

11

During the start-up phase of an investigational drug trial, you should develop a plan for managing study drug. This plan should:

1 Identify the site personnel who will receive study drug.

2 Outline the requirements for preparing and administering the drug.

3 Specify the location where study drug will be stored.

4 Determine whether there are special storage needs, such as refrigeration.

A number of factors will influence the plan, including the randomization method, the design and packaging of study drug, and the location of patients at the time study drug will be administered.

The FDA strictly mandates the labeling, packaging, shipping, and accountability of investigational drugs. The sponsor may assume these responsibilities, or may delegate responsibility to an independent agency or study pharmacy with experience in managing investigational drugs.

Study Drug Accountability

The meticulous record keeping required to track the receipt, dispensing, and final disposition of investigational drugs in clinical trials is commonly called "study drug accountability" and is necessary to document that investigational agents are administered to appropriate subjects at the assigned doses and schedules. The sponsor or study pharmacy usually supplies specific forms to aid in tracking study drug accountability, but as an investigator it is ultimately your responsibility to ensure that documentation is completed accurately and on time.

Study Drug Packaging

Study drug may be prepared and packaged in a variety of ways to maintain the study blind. Oral study drug may be supplied in blister packs, bottles, or cartons while intravenous medications may be supplied in ready-to-administer vials or in bottles with a separate vial of diluent for mixing before administration. When multiple items such as special filters or syringes are needed to prepare and administer study drug, they may be packaged with the study drug in a box or kit. A unique identifying number is generally located on the outside of the box, bottle, or vial, and the study drug box may be sealed so that it cannot be opened until assigned to a patient. In trials with blinded study drug, active drug and placebo will be packaged and labeled identically to prevent accidental or unintended breaking of the blind.

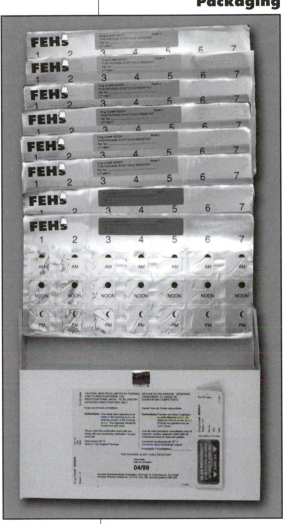

Study Drug Receipt

Study drug usually arrives at the site accompanied by a shipping invoice. When study drug supplies arrive, personnel receiving the study drug must record the date of arrival and verify that the contents of the shipment match those listed on the shipping invoice. The contents need to be examined for any broken or damaged supplies, and any

XYZ PHARMACY

FEHs
For our Examples: a Hypothetical Study

PACKING INVOICE

Site Address: _____

Pharmacy Contact: _____

Principal Investigator: _____

Shipped On: _____

BULK DRUG

Lot Number	Description	Quantity
	Total items shipped	____ vials

Please compare shipment contents to Packing Invoice. If discrepancies or damaged items are found, note on the comment line and immediately notify the XYZ Pharmacy by phone. Sign and date copies provided, return one copy to the XYZ Pharmacy and retain the other copy for your records.

Received by: _____   Date: _____

Problems Noted: _____

XYZ Pharmacy
1234 Technology Drive
Durham, NC 27704, USA
Phone: (919) 123-4567, Fax: (919) 123-3333

SITE COPY

Handling Controlled Substances

The investigator must take adequate precautions, including storage of the investigational drug in a securely locked, substantially constructed cabinet, or other securely locked, substantially constructed enclosure, access to which is limited, to prevent theft or diversion of the substance into illegal channels of distribution [21CFR § 312.69].

expiration dates must be checked. The shipment will include instructions on how to acknowledge receipt of study drug, and what should be done if there is an error on the shipping invoice or if materials are damaged. Personnel who are responsible for receiving study drug and verifying the contents should follow up on any discrepancies or concerns immediately. Keep copies of all shipping invoices and receipt acknowledgments in your site study file.

Study Drug Storage

Instructions regarding the storage of study drug and special requirements such as refrigeration at a specified temperature will be included with the shipment, in the protocol, or in a study drug reference or inservice manual. All study drug supplies must be stored in a secure location with limited access to avoid use or tampering by unauthorized personnel.

Depending on the trial, study drug may be stored in various locations at the site. For example, when patients are administered study drug in an outpatient setting, study drug should be stored in a location convenient to where the visits will be conducted. If patients are administered study drug in the emergency department, it may be beneficial to store study drug in a secure location nearby.

Dispensing Study Drug

To ensure that only enrolled patients receive study drug, you'll need a reliable system to dispense study medication. This system should take into account the individuals who will be responsible for dispensing study medication (the study coordinator or pharmacist) and the circumstances surrounding the initiation of study drug (in an acute situation such as the emergency department or a planned situation such as an outpatient clinic). The system should also provide for verifying patient eligibility for the study and, when applicable, notifying the study pharmacist when starting and stopping study drug. Every study drug kit, bottle, or vial must be accounted for to ensure that only patients involved in the study receive the investigational treatment. The sponsor or designated study pharmacy usually supplies drug accountability forms that should be updated every time study drug is dispensed to the patient or returned.

In an outpatient trial, patients may be given one or more bottles of medication to self-administer over a specified period. Instruct patients to bring their study medication to each follow-up visit so that remaining pills can be counted and returned if necessary. In a trial where intravenous drug is administered, study medication is usually recorded only as dispensed and not returned. The drug accountability forms should be designed to capture information appropriate to the specific design of the study and the study drug involved.

Study drug administration should be documented in the patient's medical record or chart as well. It is critical to carefully record study medication use as it occurs, and to sign or initial all entries on the accountability forms and in the medical record.

Control of Investigational Agents

An investigator shall administer the drug only to subjects under the investigator's personal supervision or under the supervision of a subinvestigator responsible to the investigator [21 CFR § 312.61].

FEHs

For our Examples: a Hypothetical Study

| Investigator Name: _____ | | | | | | | Protocol No.: FEHS 123-4567 |
| Patient Study No. ___ ___ ___ ___ - ___ ___ ___ | | | | | | | Drug Unblinded Yes ____ No ____ |

Drug Code No.	Visit No.	DRUG DISPENSED			DRUG RETURNED		Date/Initials Returned to Quintiles	Comments on Discrepancies	CRA Spot Checks
		No. of Caps	Date	By (initials)	No. of Caps	Counted by (initials)			

Return All Drug to:	Drug Company, Inc.	Return Shipments	1: Date Returned ___/___/___ Signed _____	
	44 Pharmaceutical Way		2: Date Returned ___/___/___ Signed _____	
	Capletville, Ohio		3: Date Returned ___/___/___ Signed _____	
	USA		4: Date Returned ___/___/___ Signed _____	

Page ____ of ____

Forms Completion
11-Jan-99
Page 12 of 12

Should You Unblind?

A patient receives an investigational drug with the potential to cause bleeding, and there is no drug known to reverse its effects. In this case, serious bleeding events should be treated by stopping ongoing study drug administration. Unblinding study treatment is not appropriate in this example, because knowing the specific agent or the dose administered would not change the treatment plan, which might include blood transfusions, pressure to the area of bleeding, and other supportive measures.

Study Drug Unblinding

There are very few appropriate reasons for breaking the study drug blind, but they include situations in which patient treatment depends on knowledge of which study drug treatment was administered.

While unblinding is a rare event, information about when and how unblinding may occur should be provided to all investigators. Methods of unblinding include tear-off labels, a telephone call to a central number, and envelopes containing the study treatment assignment or dose. Whichever method is used, remember that unblinding is appropriate in very few situations and should be carefully thought out.

Study Drug Final Disposition

The sponsor will decide if study drug or other study articles should be shipped to a designated location or destroyed at the site when the study is completed. When study drug supplies are returned to the sponsor or designated study pharmacy, have site personnel document the date, the name of the person to whom the supplies were sent, identifying information such as box or bottle numbers, and the quantity sent.

If the sponsor authorizes you to destroy study drug at the site, record the date, quantity, means of destruction, and name of the person who destroyed study drug. The final disposition of all study drug supplies should be documented on the appropriate study drug accountability forms.

"Science is organized knowledge."

—*Herbert Spencer, 19th Century British philosopher*

Patient Data Forms

12

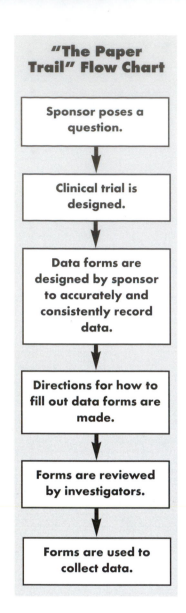

"The Paper Trail" Flow Chart

Sponsor poses a question.

↓

Clinical trial is designed.

↓

Data forms are designed by sponsor to accurately and consistently record data.

↓

Directions for how to fill out data forms are made.

↓

Forms are reviewed by investigators.

↓

Forms are used to collect data.

Clinical trials are designed to answer questions posed by the sponsor about treatment(s) identified in the protocol. To arrive at the answers to these questions, patient data are collected on forms and submitted to the sponsor or the designated data center. While the Case Report Form (CRF) is considered to be the primary data form in most trials, other data forms may be used to provide additional information important to the analysis.

Data must be reported accurately and consistently by all sites participating in the study. For this reason data forms will be reviewed carefully at investigator meetings and during monitoring visits. Directions for completing the data forms are often provided so that all sites will record data consistently using the specific definitions provided in the protocol and supplemental directions.

The nuances of the questions may not be apparent until you have had the opportunity to complete the forms for an actual patient enrolled in the study. However, a review of the data forms before the start of enrollment may help you identify protocol-related issues, procedures and logistics, such as:

1 Blood samples that are required at times different from your institution's routine

2 A physical assessment that requires an evaluation different from that routinely performed

3 Information that is not typically collected needs to be recorded

When information requested on the data forms is not typically documented in the medical records at your site, you may need to create worksheets to ensure that the data are collected and documented. Signed and dated worksheets may serve as source documentation for the data forms.

To understand the emphasis placed on data recording, data definitions, and consistency across sites, it is helpful to understand the way data are managed.

Data Management

Clinical data are collected at the investigative site, then are transferred to monitors for source document verification, to data processors for data entry and computerized checks, and finally to statisticians for analysis and reporting. The data may go back to the investigative site when the monitor needs data confirmation or correction, or when questions about the data are generated by computerized checks.

Different patterns of data flow may depend on whether data are directly entered into a computer at the investigative site, and whether monitoring and source document verification of data occurs before or after data are submitted to the data processing center.

Because computers are now so commonly used in retrieving and grouping data, data must be recorded and entered consistently. To facilitate data collection and analysis, many data forms are designed using pre-printed multiple-choice responses, with a few lines

Sample Data Form with Checkboxes and Free Text

FEHs
For our Examples: a Hypothetical Study

Patient Study Number: ___ ___ ___ - ___ ___ ___   *(site no.)*

Patient Initials: ___ ___ ___   *first middle last*

Baseline Visit

Instructions for completing this form are on the back.

Clinical History

Does the patient have a history of any of the following?

Peripheral vascular disease:	☐ No	☐ Yes
Cerebral vascular disease:	☐ No	☐ Yes
Hypertension:	☐ No	☐ Yes
Diabetes:	☐ No	☐ Yes
Severe chronic obstructive pulmonary disease:	☐ No	☐ Yes
Myocardial infarction:	☐ No	☐ Yes → If Yes, date of most recent: ___/___/___ DAY MONTH YEAR
Cardiomyopathy:	☐ No	☐ Yes → If Yes, identify type *(check one)*: ☐ Dilated ☐ Hypertrophic ☐ Other
Ejection fraction measured within the past six months:	☐ No	☐ Yes → If Yes, what is the patient's most recent EF? _____%
History of percutaneous coronary intervention:	☐ No	☐ Yes
History of CABG:	☐ No	☐ Yes
History of valvular surgery:	☐ No	☐ Yes → If Yes, check one: ☐ Mitral ☐ Aortic

Implantation Data

Date of implantation: ___/___/___ DAY MONTH YEAR

Does the patient have a sinus mechanism, a slow ectopic atrial mechanism, or atrial standstill?
☐ No → If No, patient may be ineligible. Contact Clinical Coordinating Center (305-674-2162) after implantation.
☐ Yes

Specify the lead types that are being implanted.

ATRIAL Lead *(check one)*		VENTRICULAR Lead *(check one)*	
☐ **Medtronic** →	Model #: _____	☐ **Medtronic** →	Model #: _____
☐ **Guidant** →	Model #: _____	☐ **Guidant** →	Model #: _____
☐ **Intermedics** →	Model #: _____	☐ **Intermedics** →	Model #: _____
☐ **St. Jude** →	Model #: _____	☐ **St. Jude** →	Model #: _____
☐ **Other** →	Model #: _____	☐ **Other** →	Model #: _____

183

or spaces (often referred to as "open" or "free" text) for the investigative site personnel to hand-write responses. This results in data being collected in the same terminology, and allows data to be combined easily with data from other patients and other trials.

Free Text

When free text is recorded, all terms must be consistently recorded according to the instructions. Check with the sponsor for instructions on the following situations:

1 When recording free text for an adverse event, the event should be recorded as a diagnosis or as symptoms. For example, if instructed to record a diagnosis, you should record "congestive heart failure" instead of "shortness of breath and ankle edema."

2 Although terms may be used interchangeably in clinical practice, they must be recorded consistently on data forms. For example, is "chest pain" or "ischemia" the preferred term; should "backache" or "back pain" be used?

3 When you need to record medications in a free text format instead of check boxes, ask the sponsor whether the medications should be recorded as a generic name or a trade name. For example, should you record "Lasix" or "furosemide"?

Types of Patient Data Forms

A number of data forms are listed below. This list does not include all forms, but does include many that are commonly used in clinical trials.

Enrollment Form

Enrollment forms are typically a separate worksheet used to identify and screen potential patients. The enrollment form often lists the inclusion and exclusion criteria identified in the protocol, and may be used to check off eligibility criteria as you screen the patient records. Some sponsors require the enrollment form to be submitted to the data center, while in other trials the enrollment form may be kept at the site and used as a reference and a confirmation of the screening and enrollment process.

Safety Summary Form

A safety summary form (or a similarly named form) provides a snapshot of pertinent treatment and safety information. It may be required in an inpatient trial to provide data soon after patient enrollment or after treatment with study drug or a specific intervention. Data recorded on a safety summary form are often preliminary, and may be different from the final data reported in the case report form. The data may be sent to the Data and Safety Monitoring Board to evaluate the progress of the trial, safety concerns, or treatment differences. The safety summary form is usually submitted to the data center or sponsor by fax.

Case Report Form

The Case Report Form (CRF) is the primary data form that records an enrolled patient's course of events. The CRF

FEHs
For our Examples: a Hypothetical Study

Protocol-Study #: _____ - _____
protocol number   site number
Patient's Initials: _____
first middle last

Enrollment Worksheet

Inclusion Criteria—Questions 1–4 must be answered Yes.

1 Did the patient complete A-Phase? ☐ Yes ☐ No
2 Is the patient's total cholesterol level ≤ 250 mg/dL (≤ 6.4 mmol/L)? ☐ Yes ☐ No
3 Did the patient have any of the following clinical and or angiographic risk factors? ☐ Yes ☐ No
   a. Age ≥ 70 years
   b. Diabetes mellitus (Type 1 or Type 2)
   c. Documented history of prior MI, prior CABG, prior PCI or known CAD (≥ 75% stenosis) on prior angiogram
   d. Evidence of LV dysfunction assessed by (1) ejection fraction ≤ 40%; (2) rales on clinical examination; or (3) edema on chest x-ray
   e. History of peripheral or cerebral vascular disease
   f. Additional angina with dynamic ST changes (see Study Design, Section E.1.c.1 for definition)
   g. A positive cardiac marker defined as: troponin-I or troponin-T (positive) or CK-MB > ULN or (CK ≥ 2 X ULN, if troponins or CK-MB not available) prior to any invasive procedure (catheterization or PTCA/PCI) After any invasive procedure, elevations in either troponin-I, or troponin-T or CK-MB (or CK, if troponins or CK-MB are not available) must be > 3 X ULN.
   h. A positive discharge functional study (see Study Design, Section E.1.c.2 for guidelines)
   i. Minimal coronary disease burden defined as: ≥ 2-vessel coronary artery disease (one ≥ 75% and an additional artery ≥ 50%), or single-vessel disease not revascularized
4 Was the patient clinically stable* within 120 hours of FEHs enrollment? ☐ Yes ☐ No
   *Free from the following events for 12 consecutive hours:
   a. Chest discomfort at rest
   b. Hemodynamic instability, including: systolic blood pressure < 90 mmHg for > one hour or requiring hemodynamic support, pulmonary edema, acute mitral regurgitation, or acute ventricular septal defect
   c. Ischemic events, including: recurrent symptoms of ischemia with new ST-segment or T-wave changes or reinfarction
   d. Arrhythmic events, including: ventricular fibrillation, sustained ventricular tachycardia, complete heart block, or new onset atrial fibrillation with uncontrolled ventricular rate (> 100 bpm)
   e. Miscellaneous events including: stroke, pulmonary embolus, sepsis, and acute pericarditis

Exclusion Criteria—Questions 5–8 must be answered No.

5 Further percutaneous revascularization procedures planned within the first two weeks after randomization into FEHs (i.e., PTCA/PCI) ☐ Yes ☐ No
6 No significant coronary artery disease (no lesion ≥ 75%) or single-vessel disease confirmed by diagnostic angiography, in the absence of a qualifying risk factor, when PTCA/PCI is planned either prior to or after randomization is planned? ☐ Yes ☐ No
7 CABG planned or scheduled either during or after index hospitalization, or after randomization? ☐ Yes ☐ No
8 Inability to comply with FEHs procedures? ☐ Yes ☐ No

Enrollment

Allocation # (from A-Phase): __ __ __ __   Protocol-Study #: _____ - _____   Patient's Initials: _____
                                            protocol number   site number   first middle last

Was the patient enrolled in Z-Phase? ☐ No ☐ Yes → Study Drug ID#: 5 __ __ __ __

[data management use only]

Enrollment* date and time: ___/___/___   Confirmation fax sent to site: ☐
                           day month year 00:00 to 23:59

US SITES ONLY, provide your fax #: (___) ___ - ____   Date: ___/___/___
                                                               day month year

Complete this worksheet for ALL PATIENTS and fax within 24 hours.
US: Fax to 919-123-4567 • Non-US: Fax to your local MSD office.

18 July 2000   FEHs Enrollment Worksheet, page 1 of 1

Sample Follow-up Form

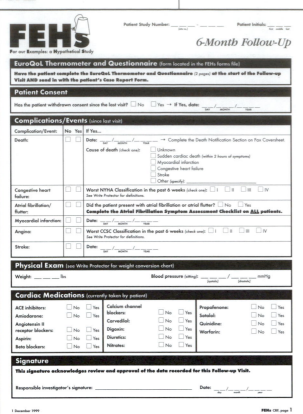

often includes information about the patient's history and pre-existing conditions in addition to events occurring at the time of and following treatment administration. The CRF may range in length from one page to more than 100 pages, depending on the complexity and requirements of a trial.

Follow-Up Forms

In some trials, follow-up forms are separate from the CRF and are used to record patient data at specified times after study enrollment, for example, at 6 months or 1 year after study enrollment. Many trials include this data as part of the CRF and do not create separate forms for follow-up data.

Serious Adverse Event Report Form

Serious Adverse Event (SAE) report forms are used to collect data pertinent to the occurrence of events that require expedited reporting to the FDA by the sponsor. Serious adverse event report forms must be reviewed and signed by the investigator, giving special attention to the description of the event and the relationship between the study treatment and the event. The sponsor, data center, or drug safety group will provide trial-specific SAE forms that should be used to report serious adverse event data. Data recorded on the final serious adverse event report forms should also be reported verbatim on the patient CRF. Refer to Chapter 5 for additional information on SAEs and general reporting requirements.

Patient-Completed Forms

Questionnaires, charts, and diaries are examples of patient-completed forms. Typically these forms are completed by patients without input from study personnel to avoid "leading" the patient to a certain response. Once the patient completes these forms, sites may be required to transcribe the patient responses onto a separate data form, or directly submit the original document completed by the patient.

FEHs
For our Examples: a Hypothetical Study

EuroQoL Questionnaire

Patient Study Number: ___ - ___ - ___   Patient Initials: ___ ___ ___
(site no.)   first middle last

EuroQoL Questionnaire

By placing a tick (✓) in one box in each group below, please indicate which statement best describes your own health state today.

Mobility:
☐ I have no problems in walking about
☐ I have some problems in walking about
☐ I am confined to bed

Self-care:
☐ I have no problems with self-care
☐ I have some problems washing or dressing myself
☐ I am unable to wash or dress myself

Usual activities (i.e. work, study, housework, family or leisure activities)**:**
☐ I have no problems with performing my usual activities
☐ I have some problems with performing my usual activities
☐ I am unable to perform my usual activities

Pain/discomfort:
☐ I have no pain or discomfort
☐ I have moderate pain or discomfort
☐ I have extreme pain or discomfort

Anxiety/depression:
☐ I am not anxious or depressed
☐ I am moderately anxious or depressed
☐ I am extremely anxious or depressed

Submitting Data

Sponsors may require that data be submitted by mail, courier, fax, or electronically via computer. The timely submission of the data is critical to meeting the deadline for data entry and analysis established by the sponsor. Instructions regarding when to submit patient data are usually provided by the sponsor or data center personnel.

Submitting Data Forms

- *Serious Adverse Event Report Forms* are usually due within 24 hours of the investigator learning of the reportable event. Serious adverse event report forms are often faxed in order to provide data to the sponsor or drug safety group within the appropriate timeframes.

- *Safety Summary Forms* are typically expected immediately after study treatment administration or upon hospital discharge. This one- to two-page form is usually submitted by fax.

- *Case Report Forms* (CRFs) may be submitted once the entire CRF is completed or at specified intervals, such as when multiple outpatient visits occur over a long period of time. When CRFs need to be verified at the site before being submitted to the data center, the monitor may be responsible for submitting the monitored CRF. In some trials the CRF is submitted to the data center without on-site data monitoring and source document verification.

- *Follow-up Forms* may be due weeks, months, or even years after the patient has completed study treatment. When follow-up forms are used, it is important to collect accurate contact information (telephone, address, name and number of relative or friend not living with patient) so that the patient can be located at the appropriate timepoints.

Submitting Data Electronically

With the increased sophistication of computers, modems, and software, some sponsors are moving toward electronic data entry by the site study personnel. This system of "remote data entry" allows the data to be directly entered into pre-designed screens at the site, bypassing the process of submitting paper copies of data forms. Data entry programs may be set up to accept only entries that fall within the protocol-specified parameters and reject entries that fall outside expected ranges. An advantage of remote data entry is the reduced time from data entry at the site to the time that data is received at the data center. Security systems, including passwords for access to data fields, are implemented to assure the integrity and confidentiality of the data, and to ensure that previously entered data are not deleted or changed. When using remote data entry, it is recommended (although not required) that a paper copy of the data forms be printed and kept at the site. The Electronic Records Rule found in Part 11 of Title 21 of the Code of Federal Regulations requires an electronic back-up of documents. The trial sponsor or data center should provide sites with specific instructions on the processes required for data back-up.

The regulations regarding electronic records and signatures can be found in 21 CFR Part 11—Electronic Records; Electronic Signatures issued in August 1997. These regulations establish the criteria under which the FDA will accept electronic records and signatures as trustworthy, reliable, and generally equivalent to paper records and handwritten signatures executed on paper. The following list summarizes some of the aspects outlined in the regulations.

1 The software used for the system must be validated. That is, its accuracy, reliability, and ability to detect invalid or altered records must have been tested and established.

2 It must be possible to generate accurate, legible copies of the electronic records, suitable for the FDA to inspect, copy, and review.

3 The records must be protected throughout the required retention period, available for accurate and ready retrieval, even if the software that created those records is no longer in use.

4 Access to the system that contains those records must be reliably limited to only authorized individuals.

5 Personnel who develop, maintain, and use these records must have documented education, training, and experience appropriate for their roles.

6 Every electronic record must have a secure, computer-generated date- and time-stamped audit trail, maintained for as long as the underlying e-record, and also available to the FDA for review and copying.

7 Reliable change control procedures, with their own time-sequenced audit trails, must be in place.

8 Written policies must exist, establishing that the record producer recognizes that anyone using an electronic signature is responsible and accountable, just as would be the case for a handwritten signature. Accompanying the signature in clear text must be the name of the signer, the date and time, and what the signature means. The system must prevent the signature from being removed, copied, or repudiated by the signer.

9 Strict requirements for passwords and other security measures must be implemented to prevent access to and falsification of e-records.

The challenge of using electronic records and signatures remains the task of creating systems and software programs that meet the regulatory requirements. However with the ever-changing technology (e.g., cell phones that access the Internet and the wide-spread use of hand-held computers), electronic records and signatures are becoming more in step with current technology and therefore more in demand by investigative sites and study subjects.

Data Form Edits and Queries

Missing values, incorrect information, and inconsistent data all represent potential sources of bias. Therefore, when the data center receives and enters the data that have been submitted by the sites, data entries that need to be edited or queried are identified. Missing responses will be requested, and data that are outside the anticipated range of answers will be explored or confirmed. Some data centers separate data questions into edits and queries, while other data centers or sponsors do not make this distinction.

Data Edits

Data edits are questions or issues identified by the data center that can be answered at the data center without sending a query to the site. An example of an edit is the insertion of a middle initial in the patient identifier when it is missing on a single data form page. Data edit changes are made at the data center and the site is notified (rather than queried) about the change. When you agree with the edit, no response may be required. However, if you disagree with the change, it is often your responsibility to respond to the data center. The data center should provide specific directions pertaining to data edits and the required action of site study personnel.

Data Queries

Data queries are questions about submitted data that require the site study staff to provide answers or clarification. Queries usually fall into one of three categories:

1 Data that are blank

2 Data that are outside a pre-specified range

3 Data that are inconsistent with other data recorded on the data forms

Reasons for Data Queries

■ *Blank Data*
To avoid unnecessary queries about blank data fields, the sponsor or data center will provide data conventions. For example, when a procedure or test was not done or there are no data to answer the question, you may be instructed to record ND in the data field. When a data question is not applicable to a particular patient or the data are not available, you may be asked to record NA in the blank.

■ *Data Outside Pre-specified Range*

Queries will be generated for data that fall outside a pre-specified or expected range. For example, if the hematocrit was recorded as 4.3 instead of 43, a query would be generated based on the expected range for hematocrit values in the study. Because ranges are established to cover both normal responses and responses slightly outside the normal range, some queries may be generated for data that were correctly recorded on the form. For example, if the pre-specified range for hematocrit values was set at 33 to 47, a hematocrit of 30 may be queried even when it was correct.

■ *Inconsistent Data*

Responses that are inconsistent with data reported elsewhere on the form will be queried. An example of inconsistent data is the reporting of a medication that was discontinued due to hypotension on one data form, yet hypotension was checked "no" elsewhere in the CRF.

Response to Data Queries

Sample Data Query Form

You may be contacted by telephone, fax, or mail to respond to data queries. Most data forms generate one or more queries that require you to review the patient records and data forms to determine if the data are correct as recorded or if they need to be changed. A response to each query should be made in a timely manner following the instructions provided. When correct data are queried, simply confirm the original value reported. To facilitate the query process, you may

FEHs Data Clarification Form

Data Clarification Form Patient Study Number: ___ ___ ___ - ___ - ___ ___ ___

To: _____   Trial Contact: _____
Phone: _____   Phone: _____
Fax: _____

For Office Use Only
Batch Date: __/__/__
Batch #: ___ ___

Data Clarification Form initiated by: ☐ Data Management ☐ CRA ☐ Site Coordinator ☐ Other: _____

Discrepancy Source	Discrepancy Message	Current Entry	Corrected Entry	F or Office Use Only
Visit/Form: Page #: Section: Item Description:				DN: VR: DU: DV: DS:
Visit/Form: Page #: Section: Item Description:				DN: VR: DU: DV: DS:

Please sign and fax to: 919-123-4567   Verified via telephone by:

_____ __/__/__   _____ __/__/__

5 November 1999   FEHs Data Clarification Form   Page 1 of 1

DN = Discrepancy Number
VR = Validation Rule
DU = Database Updated
DV = Database Verified
DS = Discrepancy Status

want to keep a copy of source documents—such as laboratory or test results—with your copies of the completed data forms.

The data center should provide instructions as to whether data changes should be made on a the specified form (such as a data query form) or directly on your copy of the CRF. Instructions for correcting data must be carefully followed so that your data forms exactly match those at the data center. Keep a copy of all corrections and query forms with the original data forms so a record or "audit trail" of changes is available.

Source Documents

Source documents are the original records of patient information. Source documents are typically signed and dated by the individual completing them and may include, but are not limited to:

1 All components of an inpatient or outpatient record

2 Consultation reports

3 Procedure and laboratory reports

4 Pharmacy records

5 Transport records, including ground and air transportation

6 Worksheets created to record pertinent data

Source Document Verification

Source documents must contain information that substantiates the data recorded on the patient data forms. An exception to this includes forms or questionnaires that are completed by patients and not transcribed by study personnel onto separate data forms. Another exception is the preliminary data recorded on a safety summary form, obtained and submitted before final data were available.

One of the primary responsibilities of the monitor during an on-site visit is to verify that data recorded on the data forms can be confirmed when compared to the source documents.

1 When erroneous data are noted on a data form or conflicting information is found in the source documents, the monitor will identify these for discussion with the site coordinator.

2 When data recorded on the forms are determined to be incorrect, the monitor will provide the site coordinator with instructions on the method and process for correcting the data.

3 When conflicting data exist within the source documents, the reasons why specific data were recorded on the forms should be documented and kept in the study file. For example, when surgery information is reported in the physician progress notes, in a surgical operative note, and in the discharge summary, it is not uncommon for minor differences to be noted. If the site coordinator or investigator knows that the most accurate and consistent information is printed in the operative note, data from that source should be recorded on the data forms and a note documenting this placed in the study file.

In some trials, source documents are submitted to the sponsor or data center for source document verification. Queries similar to those generated on-site by the monitor (based on a review of the medical record) will be sent to the site for review and response.

Release of Medical Information

In some trials, the patient may be admitted to another hospital or treated under the care of another physician. In these situations, it can be a challenge to obtain the patient's medical information. If patients will likely visit another physician or hospital, and information from those records is required in the CRF or on follow-up forms, it will be important to set up a system of medical record retrieval before study enrollment begins.

This can be accomplished by establishing a contact in the physician's office or medical record department of the patient's clinic or medical institution. You will need to determine the proper procedure for obtaining medical records from the other institutions, and obtain answers to the following questions:

1 Is there a specific form that the patient needs to sign to give you permission to obtain a copy of the records?

2 Are records available for an on-site review?

3 Does the institution charge a fee for photocopying records?

TIP: To avoid the situation where a patient is admitted to another hospital and arrangements have not been made in advance to obtain medical records from this hospital, have all study patients sign a standard *release of medical information form*. When you learn that a study patient has been admitted to another hospital or seen by another health care provider, the previously signed standard release form can be submitted to the appropriate facility. However, if the hospital or clinic requires the patient to sign a release

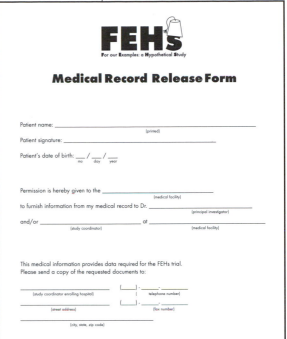

FEHs
For our Examples: a Hypothetical Study

Medical Record Release Form

Patient name: _____
 (printed)

Patient signature: _____

Patient's date of birth: ___ / ___ / ___
 mo   day   year

Permission is hereby given to the _____
 (medical facility)

to furnish information from my medical record to Dr. _____
 (principal investigator)

and/or _____ at _____
 (study coordinator)   (medical facility)

This medical information provides data required for the FEHs trial. Please send a copy of the requested documents to:

_____   (___)-_____
 (study coordinator enrolling hospital)   (telephone number)

_____   (___)-_____
 (street address)   (fax number)

_____
 (city, state, zip code)

form unique to that institution, you will need to contact the patient for a signature.

Confidentiality of Patient Information

Each clinical trial creates a system for identifying patients on the data forms. Typically, a number is assigned to the patient at the beginning of the study and is used in conjunction with the patient's initials on all forms and communication regarding the patient. Information that identifies a patient by name or provides other specific details related to patient identity should not be submitted to the sponsor or data center. When source documents such as ECGs, x-ray reports, laboratory results, and other records are submitted to the sponsor, data center, or event review committee, the patient's name and other identifying information should be crossed out or obliterated. The assigned study number and patient initials should be the only patient identifiers on the documents. Because monitors and other reviewers are permitted to see the patient's medical records on-site, it may not always be possible to maintain complete patient confidentiality. However, the patient's identity should not be apparent on the data forms or submitted source documents.

Endpoint Adjudication

Interpreting endpoint data is crucial to the analysis and reported results of a clinical trial. While investigators should follow the protocol-specified definitions when completing data forms, there may still be some variability in how investigators interpret the clinical experiences of patients enrolled in the study. Some sponsors establish an impartial group of clinicians to review endpoint data, eliminating site-to-site investigator variability. This group of clinicians, sometimes called a Clinical Endpoints Committee (CEC), reviews data forms and source documentation for specified events to determine whether an endpoint has been reached based on pre-established criteria. In the instance of a stroke, for example, the investigator may be required to send in CT and/or MRI reports and films for review by this committee. Using criteria established in the protocol, the committee reviews the films and reports, written medical records, and patient symptoms to make a decision, independently of the site investigator, about whether the endpoint was met. When the study results are published, a description of the process for reviewing and adjudicating endpoints is included.

Retention of Data Forms

Patient data forms must be kept as part of your site study file for a period of at least two years following the approval date of a New Drug Application (NDA) or two years after the sponsor notifies the FDA that the Investigational New Drug application has been discontinued. Maintaining and providing access to the records for inspection is the responsibility of the principal investigator (21 CFR § 312.62 and 312.68). Some sponsors require a longer period of record retention that may last up to 15 years for international trials. Contact the sponsor to determine the appropriate period to keep your records.

Appendices
A-F

APPENDIX A
WORLD MEDICAL ASSOCIATION
DECLARATION OF HELSINKI

Ethical Principles for
Medical Research Involving Human Subjects

Adopted by: The 18th World Medical Assembly, Helsinki, Finland, June 1964

Amended by: The 29th World Medical Assembly Tokyo, Japan, October 1975

The 35th World Medical Assembly, Venice, Italy, October 1983

The 41st World Medical Assembly, Hong Kong, September 1989

The 48th General Assembly, Somerset West, Republic of South Africa 1996

The 52nd World Medical Assembly, Edinburgh, Scotland, October 2000

A. Introduction

1.   The World Medical Association has developed the Declaration of Helsinki as a statement of ethical principles to provide guidance to physicians and other participants in medical research involving human subjects. Medical research involving human subjects includes research on identifiable human material or identifiable data.

2.   It is the duty of the physician to promote and safeguard the health of the people. The physician's knowledge and conscience are dedicated to the fulfillment of this duty.

3.   The Declaration of Geneva of the World Medical Association binds the physician with the words, "The health of my patient will be my first consideration," and the International Code of Medical Ethics declares that, "A physician shall act only in the patient's interest when providing medical care which might have the effect of weakening the physical and mental condition of the patient."

4.   Medical progress is based on research which ultimately must rest in part on experimentation involving human subjects.

5.   In medical research on human subjects, considerations related to the well-being of the human subject should take precedence over the interests of science and society.

6.   The primary purpose of medical research involving human subjects is to improve prophylactic, diagnostic and therapeutic procedures and the understanding of the etiology and pathogenesis of disease. Even the best proven prophylactic, diagnostic, and therapeutic methods must continuously be challenged through research for their effectiveness, efficiency, accessibility and quality.

7.   In current medical practice and in medical research, most prophylactic, diagnostic and therapeutic procedures involve risks and burdens.

8.   Medical research is subject to ethical standards that promote respect for all human beings and protect their health and rights. Some research populations are vulnerable and need special protection. The particular needs of the economically and medically disadvantaged must be recognized. Special attention is also required for those who cannot give or refuse consent for themselves, for those who may be subject to giving consent under duress, for those who will

not benefit personally from the research and for those for whom the research is combined with care.

9.   Research Investigators should be aware of the ethical, legal and regulatory requirements for research on human subjects in their own countries as well as applicable international requirements. No national ethical, legal or regulatory requirement should be allowed to reduce or eliminate any of the protections for human subjects set forth in this Declaration.

B. Basic Principles For All Medical Research

10.   It is the duty of the physician in medical research to protect the life, health, privacy, and dignity of the human subject.

11.   Medical research involving human subjects must conform to generally accepted scientific principles, be based on a thorough knowledge of the scientific literature, other relevant sources of information, and on adequate laboratory and, where appropriate, animal experimentation.

12.   Appropriate caution must be exercised in the conduct of research which may affect the environment, and the welfare of animals used for research must be respected.

13.   The design and performance of each experimental procedure involving human subjects should be clearly formulated in an experimental protocol. This protocol should be submitted for consideration, comment, guidance, and where appropriate, approval to a specially appointed ethical review committee, which must be independent of the investigator, the sponsor or any other kind of undue influence. This independent committee should be in conformity with the laws and regulations of the country in which the research experiment is performed. The committee has the right to monitor ongoing trials. The researcher has the obligation to provide monitoring information to the committee, especially any serious adverse events. The researcher should also submit to the committee, for review, information regarding funding, sponsors, institutional affiliations, other potential conflicts of interest and incentives for subjects.

14.   The research protocol should always contain a statement of the ethical considerations involved and should indicate that there is compliance with the principles enunciated in this Declaration.

15.   Medical research involving human subjects should be conducted only by scientifically qualified persons and under the supervision of a clinically competent medical person. The responsibility for the human subject must always rest with a medically qualified person and never rest on the subject of the research, even though the subject has given consent.

16.   Every medical research project involving human subjects should be preceded by careful assessment of predictable risks and burdens in comparison with foreseeable benefits to the subject or to others. This does not preclude the participation of healthy volunteers in medical research. The design of all studies should be publicly available.

17.   Physicians should abstain from engaging in research projects involving human subjects unless they are confident that the risks involved have been adequately assessed and can be satisfactorily managed. Physicians should cease any investigation if the risks are found to outweigh the potential benefits or if there is conclusive proof of positive and beneficial results.

18.   Medical research involving human subjects should only be conducted if the importance of the objective outweighs the inherent risks and burdens to the subject. This is especially important when the human subjects are healthy volunteers.

19.   Medical research is only justified if there is a reasonable likelihood that the populations in

which the research is carried out stand to benefit from the results of the research.

20. The subjects must be volunteers and informed participants in the research project.

21. The right of research subjects to safeguard their integrity must always be respected. Every precaution should be taken to respect the privacy of the subject, the confidentiality of the patient's information and to minimize the impact of the study on the subject's physical and mental integrity and on the personality of the subject.

22. In any research on human beings, each potential subject must be adequately informed of the aims, methods, sources of funding, any possible conflicts of interest, institutional affiliations of the researcher, the anticipated benefits and potential risks of the study and the discomfort it may entail. The subject should be informed of the right to abstain from participation in the study or to withdraw consent to participate at any time without reprisal. After ensuring that the subject has understood the information, the physician should then obtain the subject's freely-given informed consent, preferably in writing. If the consent cannot be obtained in writing, the non-written consent must be formally documented and witnessed.

23. When obtaining informed consent for the research project the physician should be particularly cautious if the subject is in a dependent relationship with the physician or may consent under duress. In that case the informed consent should be obtained by a well-informed physician who is not engaged in the investigation and who is completely independent of this relationship.

24. For a research subject who is legally incompetent, physically or mentally incapable of giving consent or is a legally incompetent minor, the investigator must obtain informed consent from the legally authorized representative in accordance with applicable law. These groups should not be included in research unless the research is necessary to promote the health of the population represented and this research cannot instead be performed on legally competent persons.

25. When a subject deemed legally incompetent, such as a minor child, is able to give assent to decisions about participation in research, the investigator must obtain that assent in addition to the consent of the legally authorized representative.

26. Research on individuals from whom it is not possible to obtain consent, including proxy or advance consent, should be done only if the physical/mental condition that prevents obtaining informed consent is a necessary characteristic of the research population. The specific reasons for involving research subjects with a condition that renders them unable to give informed consent should be stated in the experimental protocol for consideration and approval of the review committee. The protocol should state that consent to remain in the research should be obtained as soon as possible from the individual or a legally authorized surrogate.

27. Both authors and publishers have ethical obligations. In publication of the results of research, the investigators are obliged to preserve the accuracy of the results. Negative as well as positive results should be published or otherwise publicly available. Sources of funding, institutional affiliations and any possible conflicts of interest should be declared in the publication. Reports of experimentation not in accordance with the principles laid down in this Declaration should not be accepted for publication.

C. Additional Principles for Medical Research Combined with Medical Care

28. The physician may combine medical research with medical care, only to the extent that the research is justified by its potential prophylactic, diagnostic or therapeutic value. When medical research is combined with medical care, additional standards apply to protect the

patients who are research subjects.

29. The benefits, risks, burdens and effectiveness of a new method should be tested against those of the best current prophylactic, diagnostic, and therapeutic methods. This does not exclude the use of placebo, or no treatment, in studies where no proven prophylactic, diagnostic, or therapeutic method exists.

30. At the conclusion of the study, every patient entered into the study should be assured of access to the best proven prophylactic, diagnostic and therapeutic methods identified by the study.

31. The physician should fully inform the patient which aspects of the care are related to the research. The refusal of a patient to participate in a study must never interfere with the patient-physician relationship.

32. In the treatment of a patient, where proven prophylactic, diagnostic and therapeutic methods do not exist or have been ineffective, the physician, with informed consent from the patient, must be free to use unproven or new prophylactic, diagnostic and therapeutic measures, if in the physician's judgment it offers hope of saving life, re-establishing health or alleviating suffering. Where possible, these measures should be made the object of research, designed to evaluate their safety and efficacy. In all cases, new information should be recorded and, where appropriate, published. The other relevant guidelines of this Declaration should be followed.

THE BELMONT REPORT

Ethical Principles and Guidelines for the
Protection of Human Subjects of Research

The National Commission for the Protection of Human
Subjects of Biomedical and Behavioral Research
April 18, 1979

Scientific research has produced substantial social benefits. It has also posed some troubling ethical questions. Public attention was drawn to these questions by reported abuses of human subjects in biomedical experiments, especially during the Second World War. During the Nuremberg War Crime Trials, the Nuremberg code was drafted as a set of standards for judging physicians and scientists who had conducted biomedical experiments on concentration camp prisoners. This code became the prototype of many later codes[1] intended to assure that research involving human subjects would be carried out in an ethical manner.

The codes consist of rules, some general, others specific, that guide the investigators or the reviewers of research in their work. Such rules often are inadequate to cover complex situations; at times they come into conflict, and they are frequently difficult to interpret or apply. Broader ethical principles will provide a basis on which specific rules may be formulated, criticized and interpreted.

Three principles, or general prescriptive judgments, that are relevant to research involving human subjects are identified in this statement. Other principles may also be relevant. These three are comprehensive, however, and are stated at a level of generalization that should assist scientists, subjects, reviewers and interested citizens to understand the ethical issues inherent in research involving human subjects. These principles cannot always be applied so as to resolve beyond dispute particular ethical problems. The objective is to provide an analytical framework that will guide the resolution of ethical problems arising from research involving human subjects.

This statement consists of a distinction between research and practice, a discussion of the three basic ethical principles, and remarks about the application of these principles.

A. Boundaries Between Practice and Research

It is important to distinguish between biomedical and behavioral research, on the one hand, and the practice of accepted therapy on the other, in order to know what activities ought to undergo review for the protection of human subjects of research. The distinction between research and practice is blurred partly because both often occur together (as in research designed to evaluate a therapy) and partly because notable departures from standard practice are often called "experimental" when the terms "experimental" and "research" are not carefully defined.

For the most part, the term "practice" refers to interventions that are designed solely to enhance the well being of an individual patient or client and that have a reasonable expectation of success. The purpose of medical or behavioral practice is to provide diagnosis, preventive treatment or therapy to particular individuals.[2] By contrast, the term "research" designates an activity designed to test a hypothesis, permit conclusions to be drawn, and thereby to develop or contribute to generalizable knowledge (expressed, for example, in theories, principles, and statements of relationships). Research is usually described in a formal protocol that sets forth an objective and a set of procedures designed to reach that objective.

When a clinician departs in a significant way from standard or accepted practice, the innovation does not, in and of itself, constitute research. The fact that a procedure is "experimental," in the sense of new, untested or different, does not automatically place it in the category of research. Radically new procedures of this description should, however, be made the object of formal research at an early stage in order to determine whether they are safe and effective. Thus, it is the responsibility of medical practice committees, for example, to insist that a major innovation be incorporated into a formal research project.[3]

Research and practice may be carried on together when research is designed to evaluate the safety and efficacy of a therapy. This need not cause any confusion regarding whether or not the activity requires review; the general rule is that if there is any element of research in an activity, that activity should undergo review for the protection of human subjects.

B. Basic Ethical Principles

The expression "basic ethical principles" refers to those general judgments that serve as a basic justification for the many particular ethical prescriptions and evaluations of human actions. Three basic principles, among those generally accepted in our cultural tradition, are particularly relevant to the ethics of research involving human subjects: the principles of respect for persons, beneficence and justice.

1. ***Respect for Persons.*** Respect for persons incorporates at least two ethical convictions: first, that individuals should be treated as autonomous agents, and second, that persons with diminished autonomy are entitled to protection. The principle of respect for persons thus divides into two separate moral requirements: the requirement to acknowledge autonomy and the requirement to protect those with diminished autonomy.

An autonomous person is an individual capable of deliberation about personal goals and of acting under the direction of such deliberation. To respect autonomy is to give weight to autonomous persons' considered opinions and choices while refraining from obstructing their actions unless they are clearly detrimental to others. To show lack of respect for an autonomous agent is to repudiate that

206

person's considered judgments, to deny an individual the freedom to act on those considered judgments, or to withhold information necessary to make a considered judgment, when there are no compelling reasons to do so.

However, not every human being is capable of self-determination. The capacity for self-determination matures during an individual's life, and some individuals lose this capacity wholly or in part because of illness, mental disability, or circumstances that severely restrict liberty. Respect for the immature and the incapacitated may require protecting them as they mature or while they are incapacitated.

Some persons are in need of extensive protection, even to the point of excluding them from activities which may harm them; other persons require little protection beyond making sure they undertake activities freely and with awareness of possible adverse consequences. The extent of protection afforded should depend upon the risk of harm and the likelihood of benefit. The judgment that any individual lacks autonomy should be periodically reevaluated and will vary in different situations.

In most cases of research involving human subjects, respect for persons demands that subjects enter into the research voluntarily and with adequate information. In some situations, however, application of the principle is not obvious. The involvement of prisoners as subjects of research provides an instructive example. On the one hand, it would seem that the principle of respect for persons requires that prisoners not be deprived of the opportunity to volunteer for research. On the other hand, under prison conditions they may be subtly coerced or unduly influenced to engage in research activities for which they would not otherwise volunteer. Respect for persons would then dictate that prisoners be protected. Whether to allow prisoners to "volunteer" or to "protect" them presents a dilemma. Respecting persons, in most hard cases, is often a matter of balancing competing claims urged by the principle of respect itself.

2. *Beneficence.* Persons are treated in an ethical manner not only by respecting their decisions and protecting them from harm, but also by making efforts to secure their well being. Such treatment falls under the principle of beneficence. The term "beneficence" is often understood to cover acts of kindness or charity that go beyond strict obligation. In this document, beneficence is understood in a stronger sense, as an obligation. Two general rules have been formulated as complementary expressions of beneficent actions in this sense: (1) do not harm and (2) maximize possible benefits and minimize possible harms.

The Hippocratic maxim "do no harm" has long been a fundamental principle of medical ethics. Claude Bernard extended it to the realm of research, saying that one should not injure one person regardless of the benefits that might come to others. However, even avoiding harm requires learning what is harmful; and, in the process of obtaining this information, persons may be exposed to risk of harm. Further, the Hippocratic Oath requires physicians to benefit their patients "according to their best judgment." Learning what will in fact benefit may require exposing persons to risk. The problem posed by these imperatives is to decide when it is justifiable to seek certain benefits despite the risks involved, and when the benefits should be foregone because of the risks.

The obligations of beneficence affect both individual investigators and society at large, because they extend both to particular research projects and to the entire enterprise of research. In the case of particular projects, investigators and members of their institutions are obliged to give forethought to the maximization of benefits and the reduction of risk that might occur from the research investigation. In the case of scientific research in general, members of the larger society are obliged to recognize the longer term benefits and risks that may result from the improvement of knowledge and from the development of novel medical, psychotherapeutic, and social procedures.

The principle of beneficence often occupies a well-defined justifying role in many areas of research involving human subjects. An example is found in research involving children. Effective ways of treating childhood diseases and fostering healthy development are benefits that serve to justify research involving children — even when individual research subjects are not direct beneficiaries. Research also makes is possible to avoid the harm that may result from the application of previously accepted routine practices that on closer investigation turn out to be dangerous. But the role of the principle of beneficence is not always so unambiguous. A difficult ethical problem remains, for example, about research that presents more than minimal risk without immediate prospect of direct benefit to the children involved. Some have argued that such research is inadmissible, while others have pointed out that this limit would rule out much research promising great benefit to children in the future. Here again, as with all hard cases, the different claims covered by the principle of beneficence may come into conflict and force difficult choices.

3. *Justice.* Who ought to receive the benefits of research and bear its burdens? This is a question of justice, in the sense of "fairness in distribution" or "what is deserved." An injustice occurs when some benefit to which a person is entitled is denied without good reason or when some burden is imposed unduly. Another way of conceiving the principle of justice is that equals ought to be treated equally. However, this statement requires explication. Who is equal and who is unequal? What considerations justify departure from equal distribution? Almost all commentators allow that distinctions based on experience, age, deprivation, competence, merit and position do sometimes constitute criteria justifying differential treatment for certain purposes. It is necessary, then, to explain in what respects people should be treated equally. There are several widely accepted formulations of just ways to distribute burdens and benefits. Each formulation mentions some relevant property on the basis of which burdens and benefits should be distributed. These formulations are (1) to each person an equal share, (2) to each person according to individual need, (3) to each person according to individual effort, (4) to each person according to societal contribution, and (5) to each person according to merit.

Questions of justice have long been associated with social practices such as punishment, taxation and political representation. Until recently these questions have not generally been associated with scientific research. However, they are foreshadowed even in the earliest reflections on the ethics of research involving human subjects. For example, during the 19th and early 20th centuries the burdens of serving as research subjects fell largely upon poor ward patients, while the benefits of improved medical care flowed primarily to private patients. Subsequently, the exploitation of unwilling prisoners as research subjects in Nazi concentration camps was condemned as a particularly flagrant injustice. In this country, in the 1940s, the Tuskegee syphilis study used disadvantaged, rural black men to study the untreated course of a disease that is by no means confined to that population. These subjects were deprived of demonstrably effective treatment in order not to interrupt the project, long after such treatment became generally available.

Against this historical background, it can be seen how conceptions of justice are relevant to research involving human subjects. For example, the selection of research subjects needs to be scrutinized in order to determine whether some classes (e.g., welfare patients, particular racial and ethnic minorities, or persons confined to institutions) are being systematically selected simply because of their easy availability, their compromised position, or their manipulability, rather than for reasons directly related to the problem being studied. Finally, whenever research supported by public funds leads to the development of therapeutic devices and procedures, justice demands both that these not provide advantages only to those who can afford them and that such research should not unduly involve persons from groups unlikely to be among the beneficiaries of subsequent applications of the research.

C. Applications

Application of the general principles to the conduct of research leads to consideration of the following requirements: informed consent, risk/benefit assessment, and the selection of subjects of research.

1. *Informed Consent.* Respect for persons requires that subjects, to the degree that they are capable, be given the opportunity to choose what shall or shall not happen to them. This opportunity is provided when adequate standards for informed consent are satisfied.

While the importance of informed consent is unquestioned, controversy prevails over the nature and possibility of an informed consent. Nonetheless, there is widespread agreement that the consent process can be analyzed as containing three elements: information, comprehension and voluntariness.

Information. Most codes of research establish specific items for disclosure intended to assure that subjects are given sufficient information. These items generally include: the research procedure, their purposes, risks and anticipated benefits, alternative procedures (where therapy is involved), and a statement offering the subject the opportunity to ask questions and to withdraw at any time from the research. Additional items have been proposed, including how subjects are selected, the person responsible for the research, etc.

However, a simple listing of items does not answer the question of what the standard should be for judging how much and what sort of information should be provided. One standard frequently invoked in medical practice, namely the information commonly provided by practitioners in the field or in the locale, is inadequate since research takes place precisely when a common understanding does not exist. Another standard, currently popular in malpractice law, requires the practitioner to reveal the information that reasonable persons would wish to know in order to make a decision regarding their care. This, too, seems insufficient since the research subject, being in essence a volunteer, may wish to know considerably more about risks gratuitously undertaken than do patients who deliver themselves into the hand of a clinician for needed care. It may be that a standard of "the reasonable volunteer" should be proposed: the extent and nature of information should be such that persons, knowing that the procedure is neither necessary for their care nor perhaps fully understood, can decide whether they wish to participate in the furthering of knowledge. Even when some direct benefit to them is anticipated, the subjects should understand clearly the range of risk and the voluntary nature of participation.

A special problem of consent arises where informing subjects of some pertinent aspect of the research is likely to impair the validity of the research. In many cases, it is sufficient to indicate to subjects that they are being invited to participate in research of which some features will not be revealed until the research is concluded. In all cases of research involving incomplete disclosure, such research is justified only if it is clear that (1) incomplete disclosure is truly necessary to accomplish the goals of the research, (2) there are no undisclosed risks to subjects that are more than minimal, and (3) there is an adequate plan for debriefing subjects, when appropriate, and for dissemination of research results to them. Information about risks should never be withheld for the purpose of eliciting the cooperation of subjects, and truthful answers should always be given to direct questions about the research. Care should be taken to distinguish cases in which disclosure would destroy or invalidate the research from cases in which disclosure would simply inconvenience the investigator.

Comprehension. The manner and context in which information is conveyed is as important as the information itself. For example, presenting information in a disorganized and rapid fashion, allowing too little time for consideration or curtailing opportunities for questioning, all may adversely affect a subject's ability to make an informed choice.

Because the subject's ability to understand is a function of intelligence, rationality, maturity and language, it is necessary to adapt the presentation of the information to the subject's capacities.

Investigators are responsible for ascertaining that the subject has comprehended the information. While there is always an obligation to ascertain that the information about risk to subjects is complete and adequately comprehended, when the risks are more serious, that obligation increases. On occasion, it may be suitable to give some oral or written tests of comprehension.

Special provision may need to be made when comprehension is severely limited — for example, by conditions of immaturity or mental disability. Each class of subjects that one might consider as incompetent (e.g., infants and young children, mentally disabled patients, the terminally ill, and the comatose) should be considered on its own terms. Even for these persons, however, respect requires giving them the opportunity to choose to the extent they are able, whether or not to participate in research. The objections of these subjects to involvement should be honored, unless the research entails providing them a therapy unavailable elsewhere. Respect for persons also requires seeking the permission of other parties in order to protect the subjects from harm. Such persons are thus respected both by acknowledging their own wishes and by the use of third parties to protect them from harm.

The third parties chosen should be those who are most likely to understand the incompetent subject's situation and to act in that person's best interest. The person authorized to act on behalf of the subject should be given an opportunity to observe the research as it proceeds in order to be able to withdraw the subject from the research, if such action appears in the subject's best interest.

Voluntariness. An agreement to participate in research constitutes a valid consent only if voluntarily given. This element of informed consent requires conditions free of coercion and undue influence. Coercion occurs when an overt threat of harm is intentionally presented by one person to another in order to obtain compliance. Undue influence, by contrast, occurs through an offer of an excessive, unwarranted, inappropriate or improper reward or other overture in order to obtain compliance. Also, inducements that would ordinarily be acceptable may become undue influences if the subject is especially vulnerable.

Unjustifiable pressures usually occur when persons in positions of authority or commanding influence — especially where possible sanctions are involved — urge a course of action for a subject. A continuum of such influencing factors exists, however, and it is impossible to state precisely where justifiable persuasion ends and undue influence begins. But undue influence would include actions such as manipulating a person's choice through the controlling influence of a close relative and threatening to withdraw health services to which an individual would otherwise be entitled.

2. ***Assessment of Risks and Benefits.*** The assessment of risks and benefits requires a careful array of relevant data, including, in some cases, alternative ways of obtaining the benefits sought in the research. Thus, the assessment presents both an opportunity and a responsibility to gather systematic and comprehensive information about proposed research. For the investigator, it is a means to

examine whether the proposed research is properly designed. For a review committee, it is a method for determining whether the risks that will be presented to subjects are justified. For prospective subjects, the assessment will assist the determination whether or not to participate.

The Nature and Scope of Risks and Benefits. The requirement that research be justified on the basis of a favorable risk/benefit assessment bears a close relation to the principle of beneficence, just as the moral requirement that informed consent be obtained is derived primarily from the principle of respect for persons.

The term "risk" refers to a possibility that harm may occur. However, when expressions such as "small risk" or "high risk" are used, they usually refer (often ambiguously) both to the chance (probability) of experiencing a harm and the severity (magnitude) of the envisioned harm.

The term "benefit" is used in the research context to refer to something of positive value related to health or welfare. Unlike "risk," "benefit" is not a term that expresses probabilities. Risk is properly contrasted to probability of benefits, and benefits are properly contrasted with harms rather than risks of harm. Accordingly, so-called risk benefit assessments are concerned with the probabilities and magnitudes of possible harms and anticipated benefits. Many kinds of possible harms and benefits need to be taken into account. There are, for example, risks of psychological harm, physical harm, legal harm, social harm and economic harm and the corresponding benefits. While the most likely types of harms to research subjects are those of psychological or physical pain or injury, other possible kinds should not be overlooked.

Risks and benefits of research may affect the individual subjects, the families of the individual subjects, and society at large (or special groups of subjects in society). Previous codes and Federal regulations have required that risks to subjects be outweighed by the sum of both the anticipated benefit to the subject, if any, and the anticipated benefit to society in the form of knowledge to be gained from the research. In balancing these different elements, the risks and benefits affecting the immediate research subject will normally carry special weight. On the other hand, interests other than those of the subject may on some occasions be sufficient by themselves to justify the risks involved in the research, so long as the subjects' rights have been protected. Beneficence thus requires that we protect against risk of harm to subjects and also that we be concerned about the loss of the substantial benefits that might be gained from research.

The Systematic Assessment of Risks and Benefits. It is commonly said that benefits and risks must be "balanced" and shown to be "in a favorable ratio." The metaphorical character of these terms draws attention to the difficulty of making precise judgments. Only on rare occasions will quantitative techniques be available for the scrutiny of research protocols. However, the idea of systematic, non-arbitrary analysis of risks and benefits should be emulated insofar as possible. This ideal requires those making decisions about the justifiability of research to be thorough in the accumulation and assessment of information about all aspects of the research, and to consider alternatives systematically. This procedure renders the assessment of research more rigorous and precise, while making communication between review board members and investigators less subject to misinterpretation, misinformation and conflicting judgments. Thus, there should first be a determination of the validity of the presuppositions of the research; then the nature, probability and magnitude of risk should be distinguished with as much clarity as possible. The method of ascertaining risks should be explicit, especially where there is no alternative to the use of such vague categories as small or slight risk. It should also be determined whether an investigator's estimates of the probability of harm or benefits are reasonable, as judged by known facts or other available studies.

Finally, assessment of the justifiability of research should reflect at least the following considerations: (i) Brutal or inhumane treatment of human subjects is never morally justified. (ii) Risks should be reduced to those necessary to achieve the research objective. It should be determined whether it is in fact necessary to use human subjects at all. Risk can perhaps never be entirely eliminated, but it can often be reduced by careful attention to alternative procedures. (iii) When research involves significant risk of serious impairment, review committees should be extraordinarily insistent on the justification of the risk (looking usually to the likelihood of benefit to the subject or, in some rare cases, to the manifest voluntariness of the participation). (iv) When vulnerable populations are involved in research, the appropriateness of involving them should itself be demonstrated. A number of variables go into such judgments, including the nature and degree of risk, the condition of the particular population involved, and the nature and level of the anticipated benefits. (v) Relevant risks and benefits must be thoroughly arrayed in documents and procedures used in the informed consent process.

3. *Selection of Subjects.* Just as the principle of respect for persons finds expression in the requirements for consent and the principle of beneficence in risk benefit assessment, the principle of justice gives rise to moral requirements that there be fair procedures and outcomes in the selection of research subjects.

Justice is relevant to the selection of subjects of research at two levels: the social and the individual. Individual justice in the selection of subjects would require that researchers exhibit fairness: thus, they should not offer potentially beneficial research only to some patients who are in their favor or select only "undesirable" persons for risky research. Social justice requires that distinction be drawn between classes of subjects that ought, and ought not, to participate in any particular kind of research, based on the ability of members of that class to bear burdens and on the appropriateness of placing further burdens on already burdened persons. Thus, it can be considered a matter of social justice that there is an order of preference in the selection of classes of subjects (e.g., adults before children) and that some classes of potential subjects (e.g., the institutionalized mentally infirm or prisoners) may be involved as research subjects, if at all, only on certain conditions.

Injustice may appear in the selection of subjects, even if individual subjects are selected fairly by investigators and treated fairly in the course of research. Thus injustice arises from social, racial, sexual, and cultural biases institutionalized in society. Thus, even if individual researchers are treating their research subjects fairly, and even if IRBs are taking care to assure that subjects are selected fairly within a particular institution, unjust social patterns may nevertheless appear in the overall distribution of the burdens and benefits of research. Although individual institutions or investigators may not be able to resolve a problem that is pervasive in their social setting, they can consider distributive justice in selecting research subjects.

Some populations, especially institutionalized ones, are already burdened in many ways by their infirmities and environments. When research is proposed that involves risks and does not include a therapeutic component, other less burdened classes of persons should be called upon first to accept these risks of research, except where the research is directly related to the specific conditions of the class involved. Also, even though public funds for research may often flow in the same directions as public funds for health care, it seems unfair that populations dependent on public health care constitute a pool of preferred research subjects if more advantaged populations are likely to be the recipients of the benefits.

One special instance of injustice results from the involvement of vulnerable subjects. Certain groups, such as racial minorities, the economically disadvantaged, the very sick, and the institutionalized may continually be sought as research subjects, owing to their ready availability in settings where research is conducted. Given their dependent status and their frequently compromised capacity for free consent, they should be protected against the danger of being involved in research solely for administrative convenience, or because they are easy to manipulate as a result of their illness or socioeconomic condition.

Appendix B
Sample Template for a Consent Form
Consent to Participate in a Research Study

> Text within boxes in each section refers to the basic and additional informed consent elements in the Code of Federal Regulations (21 § CFR 50.25).

Protocol Number/Study Title:

Principal Investigator:

Name of Site (or sites) of Investigation:

Introduction

You are being asked to participate in a research study. Before you give your consent to participate, read the following information and ask as many questions as necessary to be sure you understand what your participation involves.

Background Information and Purpose of the Study

> *Basic Element:* Informed consent must include a statement that the study involves research, an explanation of the purpose of the research, and the expected duration of the subject's participation.

You are being asked to participate in a research study to evaluate (*describe purpose in lay terms and identify study drug, device or procedure as investigational*). This study is being conducted because (*provide background information*).

> *Additional Element:* When appropriate, informed consent must include the approximate number of subjects involved in the study.

Approximately *XX* subjects will be enrolled in this study at *XX* sites in the United States over a period of *XX*.

Study Procedures

> *Basic Element:* Informed consent must include a description of the procedures to be followed and identification of procedures that are experimental.

If you agree to participate in this study, the following procedures will be performed (*list and describe study procedures*):

Example: You will be assigned to receive either a dose of study medication or a placebo (inactive substance). Neither you nor your doctor will know which you are receiving. There is a 2 in 3 chance that you will receive the study medication and a 1 out of 3 chance that you will receive placebo.

Foreseeable Risks or Discomforts

> *Basic Element:* Informed consent must include a description of reasonably foreseeable risks or discomforts.

There are some possible risks or discomforts that might occur as a result of the above mentioned study procedures. (*In lay language, identify side effects associated with the use of the investigational treatment and risks that may result from research related tests and procedures.*) Potential risks or discomforts include:

Example: Having your blood drawn is momentarily uncomfortable. There is a small risk of bruising and a rare risk of infection (1/1000 chance) at the site where the blood is drawn.

> *Additional Element:* When appropriate, informed consent must include a statement that the particular treatment or procedure may involve risks to the subject (or to the embryo or fetus, if the subject is or may become pregnant) which are currently unforeseeable.

In addition to the risks listed above, there may be other risks that are currently not foreseeable. These could include risks to you or to your embryo or fetus should you become pregnant.

> *Additional Element*: When appropriate, informed consent must include a statement that significant new findings developed during the course of the research which may relate to the subject's willingness to continue participation will be provided to the subject.

Any significant new findings that develop during the course of the study that may affect your willingness to continue participation will be provided to you.

Benefits

> *Basic Element:* Informed consent must include a description of any benefits to the subject or to others that may reasonably be expected from the research.

It is not known whether you will personally benefit as a result of your participation in this study. Benefits might include (*describe possible benefits*):

Example: The study medication may (*describe the desired effect e.g., reduce the size of your tumor*).

While it is possible that you will not obtain any benefits from participating, the information gained through your involvement may help others with the same health condition in the future.

Alternative Treatment

> *Basic Element*: Informed consent must include a disclosure of appropriate alternative procedures or courses of treatment, if any, that might be advantageous to the subject.

There are other treatments available for (*identify disease condition being evaluated*). These treatments include (*list possible treatments*):

Example: If you do not participate in the study, you will probably be given (*name of non-study medication*).

If you decide not to participate in this study, you and your physician will discuss what treatments would best meet your needs. If you choose to be in the study, you may stop your participation at any time without jeopardy to your medical care.

Compensation for Participation

> *Additional Element*: When appropriate, informed consent must include a description of additional costs to the subject that may result from participation in the research.

There is no money paid to you for participating in this study; however, you will not have to pay for the tests and procedures that are done specifically for this research study. You will not be billed for (*list study procedures that are paid for out of study budget*). Procedures that would be done as part of the routine care for your health condition will be billed to you or your insurance carrier as usual. Any other costs related to the care or treatment of your health condition will be your financial responsibility.

Compensation for Research-Related Injury

> *Basic Element:* When research involves more than minimal risk, informed consent must include an explanation as to whether compensation and medical treatments are available if injury occurs, and if so, what they consist of or where further information may be obtained.

Every effort to prevent injury that could result from this study will be taken; however, if you are injured as a result of your participation, immediate necessary care will be provided to you. _____ , the sponsor of this study (will/will not) provide financial payment for reasonable medical expenses that occur as a direct result of the study treatment. The availability of this compensation may depend upon the circumstances involved, and there are limitations that may apply. For general information about compensation for research-related injuries, you may contact _____ (IRB contact) at ___ - ___-_____ (phone). You should notify _____ (investigator) at ___ - ___-_____ (phone) immediately if any new condition or injury develops during the course of this study, or if you need specific information about medical treatment for a study-related injury.

Withdrawal from the Study

> *Basic Element:* Informed consent must include a statement that research is voluntary, and that refusal to participate or discontinuation of participation will not involve any penalty or loss of benefits to which the subject is otherwise entitled.

Your participation in this study is completely voluntary. You have the right to refuse to participate or to withdraw at any time without jeopardy to your health care.

> *Additional Element:* When appropriate, informed consent must include a statement of the consequences of a subject's decision to withdraw from the research and procedures for orderly termination of participation by the subject.

If you decide to stop participation at any time, contact _____ (investigator) at ___ - ___-_____ (phone) to inform him/her of your decision and decide how best to proceed with your medical care.

Your participation in the study may be stopped by _____ (investigator) if it is determined to be in your best interest to do so.

Release of Medical Records and Confidentiality

All information about you will be held confidential. The study personnel at this institution, the sponsor of the study, reviewers designated by the sponsor, and the Food and Drug Administration will have access to your medical records for review of study information. Your records will be handled as confidentially as is possible. If the results of this study are reported in medical journals or at medical meetings, your identity will remain confidential.

Contact Information

For answers to questions about this research study, to report a research-related injury, or for information regarding study procedures you may contact _____ (investigator) at ___-___-_____ (phone).

This consent form and research study have been reviewed by the Investigational Review Board. If you have questions regarding your rights as a research study participant, you may contact _____ (IRB contact) at ___-___-_____ (phone).

Consent to Participate

Your signature below indicates that you have chosen to participate in this research study. You will be given a copy of this consent form to keep.

_____   _____
       Signature Subject/Patient (or legal guardian)   Date

_____
       Printed Subject/Patient Name (or legal guardian)

To the best of my knowledge, the subject/patient signing this consent form understands the nature, risks, and benefits of this research study and voluntarily agrees to participate.

_____   _____
       Signature of Person Obtaining Consent   Date

218

Appendix C

Code of Federal Regulations

The Code of Federal Regulations contains laws that regulate the conduct of clinical trials. Below are some of the regulations excerpted from the Code of Federal Regulations (CFR) revised April 1, 2000, that pertain to financial disclosure for investigators participating in clinical studies and to responsibilities of site investigators, investigational review boards, and sponsors of clinical trials. For a comprehensive review of all the regulations, refer to the most current and complete version of the regulations. Title 21 regulations are revised and published annually on April 1st; Title 45 regulations are revised and published annually on October 1st. Between annual publications, the CFR is kept up to date by individual issues of the Federal Register. The CFR and the Federal Register should be used together to determine the latest version of any rule.

The regulations in Parts 50 (Protection of Human Subjects), 54 (Financial Disclosure by Clinical Investigators), and 56 (Institutional Review Boards) apply to all clinical trials. Regulations excerpted from Parts 312 (Investigational New Drug Application) and 314 (Application For FDA Approval to Market a New Drug) apply to investigational drugs, and those from Parts 812 (Investigational Device Exemptions) and 814 (Premarket Approval of Medical Devices) to medical devices.

Sections of the Code of Federal Regulations that are not reproduced here can be found at http://www.access.gpo.gov/nara/cfr/cfr-table-search.html.

Regulations Affecting Investigators

21 CFR § 312.60 General responsibilities of investigators (investigational drugs)
An investigator is responsible for ensuring that an investigation is conducted according to the signed investigator statement, the investigational plan, and applicable regulations; for protecting the rights, safety, and welfare of subjects under the investigator's care; and for the control of drugs under investigation. An investigator shall, in accordance with the provisions of part 50 of this chapter, obtain the informed consent of each human subject to whom the drug is administered, except as provided in §50.23 or §50.24 of this chapter. Additional specific responsibilities of clinical investigators are set forth in this part and in parts 50 and 56 of this chapter.

21 CFR § 812.100 General responsibilities of investigators (medical devices)
An investigator is responsible for ensuring that an investigation is conducted according to the signed agreement, the investigational plan and applicable FDA regulations, for protecting the rights, safety, and welfare of subjects under the investigator's care, and for the control of devices under investigation. An investigator also is responsible for ensuring that informed consent is obtained in accordance with part 50 of this chapter. Additional responsibilities of investigators are described in subpart G.

21 CFR § 312.61 Control of the investigational drug (investigational drugs)

An investigator shall administer the drug only to subjects under the investigator's personal supervision or under the supervision of a subinvestigator responsible to the investigator. The investigator shall not supply the investigational drug to any person not authorized under this part to receive it.

21 CFR § 312.62 Investigator recordkeeping and record retention (investigational drugs)

(a) *Disposition of drug.* An investigator is required to maintain adequate records of the disposition of the drug, including dates, quantity, and use by subjects. If the investigation is terminated, suspended, discontinued, or completed, the investigator shall return the unused supplies of the drug to the sponsor, or otherwise provide for disposition of the unused supplies of the drug under §312.59.

(b) *Case histories.* An investigator is required to prepare and maintain adequate and accurate case histories designed to record all observations and other data pertinent to the investigation on each individual administered the investigational drug or employed as a control in the investigation. Case histories include the case report forms and supporting data including, for example, signed and dated consent forms, any medical records, for example, progress notes of the physician, the individual's hospital chart(s), and nurses' notes. The case history for each individual shall document that informed consent was obtained prior to participation in the study.

(c) *Record retention.* An investigator shall retain records required to be maintained under this part for a period of 2 years following the date a marketing application is approved for the drug for the indication for which it is being investigated; or, if no application is to be filed or if the application is not approved for such indication, until 2 years after the investigation is discontinued and FDA is notified.

21 CFR § 312.64 Investigator reports (investigational drugs)

(a) *Progress reports.* The investigator shall furnish all reports to the sponsor of the drug who is responsible for collecting and evaluating the results obtained. The sponsor is required under §312.33 to submit annual reports to FDA on the progress of clinical investigations.

(b) *Safety reports.* An investigator shall promptly report to the sponsor any adverse effect that may reasonably be regarded as caused by, or probably caused by, the drug. If the adverse effect is alarming, the investigator shall report the adverse effect immediately.

(c) *Final report.* An investigator shall provide the sponsor with an adequate report shortly after completion of the investigator's participation in the investigation.

(d) *Financial disclosure reports.* The clinical investigator shall provide the sponsor with sufficient accurate financial information to allow an applicant to submit complete and accurate certification or disclosure statements as required under part 54 of this chapter. The clinical investigator shall promptly update this information if any relevant changes occur during the course of the investigation and for 1 year following the completion of the study.

21 CFR § 812.150 Reports (medical devices)

(a) *Investigator reports.* An investigator shall prepare and submit the following complete, accurate, and timely reports:

      (1) *Unanticipated adverse device effects.* An investigator shall submit to the sponsor and to the reviewing IRB a report of any unanticipated adverse device effect occurring during

an investigation as soon as possible, but in no event later than 10 working days after the investigator first learns of the effect.

(2) *Withdrawal of IRB approval.* An investigator shall report to the sponsor, within 5 working days, a withdrawal of approval by the reviewing IRB of the investigator's part of an investigation.

(3) *Progress.* An investigator shall submit progress reports on the investigation to the sponsor, the monitor, and the reviewing IRB at regular intervals, but in no event less often than yearly.

(4) *Deviations from the investigational plan.* An investigator shall notify the sponsor and the reviewing IRB of any deviation from the investigational plan to protect the life or physical well-being of a subject in an emergency. Such notice shall be given as soon as possible, but in no event later than 5 working days after the emergency occurred. Except in such an emergency, prior approval by the sponsor is required for changes in or deviations from a plan, and if these changes or deviations may affect the scientific soundness of the plan or the rights, safety, or welfare of human subjects, FDA and IRB in accordance with § 812.35(a) also is required.

(5) *Informed consent.* If an investigator uses a device without obtaining informed consent, the investigator shall report such use to the sponsor and the reviewing IRB within 5 working days after the use occurs.

(6) *Final report.* An investigator shall within 3 months after termination or completion of the investigation or the investigator's part of the investigation, submit a final report to the sponsor and the reviewing IRB.

(7) *Other.* An investigator shall, upon request by a reviewing IRB or FDA, provide accurate, complete, and current information about any aspect of the investigation.

21 CFR § 312.66 Assurance of IRB review (investigational drugs)
An investigator shall assure that an IRB that complies with the requirements set forth in Part 56 will be responsible for the initial and continuing review and approval of the proposed clinical study. The investigator shall also assure that he or she will promptly report to the IRB all changes in the research activity and all unanticipated problems involving risk to human subjects or others, and that he or she will not make any changes in the research without IRB approval, except where necessary to eliminate apparent immediate hazards to human subjects.

21 CFR § 312.68 Inspection of investigator's records and reports (investigational drugs)
An investigator shall upon request from any properly authorized officer or employee of FDA, at reasonable times, permit such officer or employee to have access to, and copy and verify any records or reports made by the investigator pursuant to §312.62. The investigator is not required to divulge subject names unless the records of particular individuals require a more detailed study of the cases, or unless there is reason to believe that the records do not represent actual case studies, or do not represent actual results obtained.

21 CFR § 312.69 Handling of controlled substances (investigational drugs)
If the investigational drug is subject to the Controlled Substances Act, the investigator shall take adequate precautions, including storage of the investigational drug in a securely locked, substantially constructed cabinet, or other securely locked, substantially constructed enclosure, access to which is limited, to prevent theft or diversion of the substance into illegal channels of distribution.

21 CFR § 50.20 General requirements for informed consent (human subjects protection)
Except as provided in §50.23 and §50.24, no investigator may involve a human being as a subject in research covered by these regulations unless the investigator has obtained the legally effective

informed consent of the subject or the subject's legally authorized representative. An investigator shall seek such consent only under circumstances that provide the prospective subject or the representative sufficient opportunity to consider whether or not to participate and that minimize the possibility of coercion or undue influence. The information that is given to the subject or the representative shall be in language understandable to the subject or the representative. No informed consent, whether oral or written, may include any exculpatory language through which the subject or the representative is made to waive or appear to waive any of the subject's legal rights, or releases or appears to release the investigator, the sponsor, the institution, or its agents from liability for negligence.

21 CFR § 50.25 Elements of informed consent (human subjects protection)

(a) *Basic elements of informed consent.* In seeking informed consent, the following information shall be provided to each subject:

> (1) A statement that the study involves research, an explanation of the purposes of the research and the expected duration of the subject's participation, a description of the procedures to be followed, and identification of any procedures which are experimental.
> (2) A description of any reasonably foreseeable risks or discomforts to the subject.
> (3) A description of any benefits to the subject or to others which may reasonably be expected from the research.
> (4) A disclosure of appropriate alternative procedures or courses of treatment, if any, that might be advantageous to the subject.
> (5) A statement describing the extent, if any, to which confidentiality of records identifying the subject will be maintained and that notes the possibility that the Food and Drug Administration may inspect the records.
> (6) For research involving more than minimal risk, an explanation as to whether any compensation and an explanation as to whether any medical treatments are available if injury occurs and, if so, what they consist of, or where further information may be obtained.
> (7) An explanation of whom to contact for answers to pertinent questions about the research and research subject's rights, and whom to contact in the event of a research-related injury to the subject.
> (8) A statement that participation is voluntary, that refusal to participate will involve no penalty or loss of benefits to which the subject is otherwise entitled, and that the subject may discontinue participation at any time without penalty or loss of benefits to which the subject is otherwise entitled.

(b) *Additional elements of informed consent.* When appropriate, one or more of the following elements of information shall also be provided to each subject:

> (1) A statement that the particular treatment or procedure may involve risks to the subject (or to the embryo or fetus, if the subject is or may become pregnant) which are currently unforeseeable.
> (2) Anticipated circumstances under which the subject's participation may be terminated by the investigator without regard to the subject's consent.
> (3) Any additional costs to the subject that may result from participation in the research.
> (4) The consequences of a subject's decision to withdraw from the research and procedures for orderly termination of participation by the subject.
> (5) A statement that significant new findings developed during the course of the research which may relate to the subject's willingness to continue participation will be provided to the subject.
> (6) The approximate number of subjects involved in the study.

(c)   The informed consent requirements in these regulations are not intended to preempt any applicable Federal, State, or local laws which require additional information to be disclosed for informed consent to be legally effective.

(d)   Nothing in these regulations is intended to limit the authority of a physician to provide emergency medical care to the extent the physician is permitted to do so under applicable Federal, State, or local law.

21 CFR § 50.27 Documentation of informed consent (human subjects protection)

(a)   Except as provided in §56.109 (c), informed consent shall be documented by the use of a written consent form approved by the IRB and signed and dated by the subject or the subject's legally authorized representative at the time of consent. A copy shall be given to the person signing the form.

(b)   Except as provided in §56.109 (c), the consent form may be either of the following:

(1) A written consent document that embodies the elements of informed consent required by §50.25. This form may be read to the subject or the subject's legally authorized representative, but, in any event, the investigator shall give either the subject or the representative adequate opportunity to read it before it is signed.

(2) A *short form* written consent document stating that the elements of informed consent required by §50.25 have been presented orally to the subject or the subject's legally authorized representative. When this method is used, there shall be a witness to the oral presentation. Also, the IRB shall approve a written summary of what is to be said to the subject or the representative. Only the short form itself is to be signed by the subject or the representative. However, the witness shall sign both the short form and a copy of the summary, and the person actually obtaining the consent shall sign a copy of the summary. A copy of the summary shall be given to the subject or the representative in addition to a copy of the short form.

Regulations Affecting Institutional Review Boards

21 CFR § 56.107 IRB membership

(a)   Each IRB shall have at least five members, with varying backgrounds to promote complete and adequate review of research activities commonly conducted by the institution. The IRB shall be sufficiently qualified through the experience and expertise of its members, and the diversity of the members, including consideration of race, gender, cultural backgrounds, and sensitivity to such issues as community attitudes, to promote respect for its advice and counsel in safeguarding the rights and welfare of human subjects. In addition to possessing the professional competence necessary to review the specific research activities, the IRB shall be able to ascertain the acceptability of proposed research in terms of institutional commitments and regulations, applicable law, and standards or professional conduct and practice. The IRB shall therefore include persons knowledgeable in these areas. If an IRB regularly reviews research that involves a vulnerable category of subjects, such as children, prisoners, pregnant women, or handicapped or mentally disabled persons, consideration shall be given to the inclusion of one or more individuals who are knowledgeable about and experienced in working with those subjects.

(b)   Every nondiscriminatory effort will be made to ensure that no IRB consists entirely of men or entirely of women, including the institution's consideration of qualified persons of both sexes, so long as no selection is made to the IRB on the basis of gender. No IRB may consist entirely

Appendix C

of members of one profession.

(c)   Each IRB shall include at least one member whose primary concerns are in the scientific area and at least one member whose primary concerns are in nonscientific areas.

(d)   Each IRB shall include at least one member who is not otherwise affiliated with the institution and who is not part of the immediate family of a person who is affiliated with the institution.

(e)   No IRB may have a member participate in the IRB's initial or continuing review of any project in which the member has a conflicting interest, except to provide information requested by the IRB.

(f)   An IRB may, in its discretion, invite individuals with competence in special areas to assist in the review of complex issues which require expertise beyond or in addition to that available on the IRB. These individuals may not vote with the IRB.

21 CFR § 56.109 IRB review of research

(a)   An IRB shall review and have authority to approve, require modifications in (to secure approval), or disapprove all research activities covered by these regulations.

(b)   An IRB shall require that information given to subjects as part of informed consent is in accordance with §50.25. The IRB may require that information, in addition to that specifically mentioned in §50.25, be given to the subjects when in the IRB's judgment the information would meaningfully add to the protection of the rights and welfare of subjects.

(c)   An IRB shall require documentation of informed consent in accordance with §50.27 of this chapter, except as follows:
(1) the IRB may, for some or all subjects, waive the requirement that the subject or the subject's legally authorized representative sign a written consent form if it finds that the research presents no more than minimal risk of harm to subjects and involves no procedures for which written consent is normally required outside the research context, or
(2) The IRB may, for some or all subjects, find that the requirements in §50.24 of this chapter for an exception from informed consent for emergency research are met.

(d)   In cases where the documentation requirement is waived under paragraph (c)(1) of this section, the IRB may require the investigator to provide subjects with a written statement regarding the research.

(e)   An IRB shall notify investigators and the institution in writing of its decision to approve or disapprove the proposed research activity, or of modifications required to secure IRB approval of the research activity. If the IRB decides to disapprove a research activity, it shall include in its written notification a statement of the reasons for its decision and give the investigator an opportunity to respond in person or in writing. For investigations involving an exception to informed consent under §50.24 of this chapter, an IRB shall promptly notify in writing the investigator and the sponsor of the research when an IRB determines that it cannot approve the research because it does not meet the criteria in the exception provided under §50.24(a) of this chapter or because of other relevant ethical concerns. The written notification shall include a statement of the reasons for the IRB's determination.

(f)   An IRB shall conduct continuing review of research covered by these regulations at intervals appropriate to the degree of risk, but not less than once per year, and shall have authority to observe or have a third party observe the consent process and the research.

(g)   An IRB shall provide in writing to the sponsor of research involving an exception to informed

consent under §50.24 of this chapter a copy of information that has been publicly disclosed under §50.24(a)(7)(ii) and (a)(7)(iii) of this chapter. The IRB shall provide this information to the sponsor promptly so that the sponsor is aware that such disclosure has occurred. Upon receipt, the sponsor shall provide copies of the information disclosed to the FDA.

21 CFR § 56.110 Expedited review procedures for certain kinds of research involving no more than minimal risk, and for minor changes in approved research.

(a) The Food and Drug Administration has established, and published in the Federal Register, a list of categories of research that may be reviewed by the IRB through an expedited review procedure. The list will be amended, as appropriate, through periodic republication in the Federal Register.

(b) An IRB may use the expedited review procedure to review either or both of the following: (1) Some or all of the research appearing on the list and found by the reviewer(s) to involve no more than minimal risk, (2) minor changes in previously approved research during the period (of 1 year or less) for which approval is authorized. Under an expedited review procedure, the review may be carried out by the IRB chairperson or by one or more experienced reviewers designated by the IRB chairperson from among the members of the IRB. In reviewing the research, the reviewers may exercise all of the authorities of the IRB except that the reviewers may not disapprove the research. A research activity may be disapproved only after review in accordance with the nonexpedited review procedure set forth in §56.108(c).

(c) Each IRB which uses an expedited review procedure shall adopt a method for keeping all members advised of research proposals which have been approved under the procedure.

(d) The Food and Drug Administration may restrict, suspend, or terminate an institution's or IRB's use of the expedited review procedure when necessary to protect the rights or welfare of subjects.

Regulations Affecting Sponsors

21 CFR § 312.50 General responsibilities of sponsors (investigational drugs)
Sponsors are responsible for selecting qualified investigators, providing them with the information they need to conduct an investigation properly, ensuring proper monitoring of the investigation(s), ensuring that the investigation(s) is conducted in accordance with the general investigational plan and protocols contained in the IND, maintaining an effective IND with respect to the investigations, and ensuring that FDA and all participating investigators are promptly informed of significant new adverse effects or risks with respect to the drug. Additional specific responsibilities of sponsors are described elsewhere in this part.

21 CFR § 812.40 General responsibilities of sponsors (medical devices)
Sponsors are responsible for selecting qualified investigators and providing them with the information they need to conduct the investigation properly, ensuring proper monitoring of the investigation, ensuring that IRB review and approval are obtained, submitting an IDE application to FDA, and ensuring that any reviewing IRB and FDA are promptly informed of significant new information about an investigation. Additional responsibilities of sponsors are described in subparts B and G.

Appendix C

21 CFR § 312.52 Transfer of obligations to a contract research organization *(investigational drugs)

(a)   A sponsor may transfer responsibility for any or all of the obligations set forth in this part to a contract research organization. Any such transfer shall be described in writing. If not all obligations are transferred, the writing is required to describe each of the obligations being assumed by the contract research organization. If all obligations are transferred, a general statement that all obligations have been transferred is acceptable. Any obligation not covered by the written description shall be deemed not to have been transferred.

(b)   A contract research organization that assumes any obligation of a sponsor shall comply with the specific regulations in this chapter applicable to this obligation and shall be subject to the same regulatory action as a sponsor for failure to comply with any obligation assumed under these regulations. Thus, all references to "sponsor" in this part apply to a contract research organization to the extent that it assumes one or more obligations of the sponsor.

21 CFR § 312.53 Selecting investigators and monitors (investigational drugs)

(a)   *Selecting investigators.* A sponsor shall select only investigators qualified by training and experience as appropriate experts to investigate the drug.

(b)   *Control of drug.* A sponsor shall ship investigational new drugs only to investigators participating in the investigation.

(c)   *Obtaining information from the investigator.* Before permitting an investigator to begin participation in an investigation, the sponsor shall obtain the following:

(1) A signed investigator statement (Form FDA-1572). *Additional details in the regulations.*
(2) Curriculum Vitae. A curriculum vitae or other statement of qualifications of the investigator showing the education, training, and experience that qualifies the investigator as an expert in the clinical investigation of the drug for the use under investigation.
(3) Clinical protocol. (i) For Phase 1 investigations a general outline of the planned investigation including the estimated duration of the study and the maximum number of subjects that will be involved. (ii) For Phase 2 or 3 investigations, an outline of the study protocol including an approximation of the number of subjects to be treated with the drug and the number to be employed as controls, if any; the clinical uses to be investigated; characteristics of subjects by age, sex, and condition; the kind of clinical observations and laboratory tests to be conducted; the estimated duration of the study; and copies or a description of case report forms to be used.
(4) Financial disclosure information. Sufficient accurate financial information to allow the sponsor to submit complete and accurate certification of disclosure statements required under part 54 of this chapter. The sponsor shall obtain a commitment from the clinical investigator to promptly update this information if any relevant changes occur during the course of the investigation and for 1 year following the completion of the study.

(d)   *Selecting monitors.* A sponsor shall select a monitor qualified by training and experience to monitor the progress of the investigation.

21 CFR § 312.55 Informing investigators (investigational drugs)

(a)   Before the investigation begins, a sponsor (other than a sponsor-investigator) shall give each participating clinical investigator an investigator brochure containing the information described in §312.23 (a)(5).

(b) The sponsor shall, as the overall investigation proceeds, keep each participating investigator informed of new observations discovered by or reported to the sponsor on the drug, particularly with respect to adverse effects and safe use. Such information may be distributed to investigators by means of periodically revised investigator brochures, reprints or published studies, reports or letters to clinical investigators, or other appropriate means. Important safety information is required to be relayed to investigators in accordance with §312.32.

21 CFR § 312.56 Review of ongoing investigations (investigational drugs)

(a) The sponsor shall monitor the progress of all clinical investigations being conducted under its IND.

(b) A sponsor who discovers that an investigator is not complying with the signed agreement (Form FDA-1572), the general investigational plan, or the requirements of this part or other applicable parts shall promptly either secure compliance or discontinue shipments of the investigational new drug to the investigator and end the investigator's participation in the investigation. If the investigator's participation is ended, the sponsor shall require that the investigator dispose of or return the investigational drug in accordance with the requirements of §312.59 and shall notify the FDA.

(c) The sponsor shall review and evaluate the evidence relating to the safety and effectiveness of the drug as it is obtained from the investigator. The sponsors shall make such reports to FDA regarding information relevant to the safety of the drug as are required under §312.32. The sponsor shall make annual reports on the progress of the investigation in accordance with §312.33.

(d) A sponsor who determines that its investigational drug presents an unreasonable and significant risk to subjects shall discontinue those investigations that present the risk, notify FDA, all institutional review boards, and all investigators who have at any time participated in the investigation of the discontinuance, assure the disposition of all stocks of the drug outstanding as required by §312.59, and furnish FDA with a full report of the sponsor's actions. The sponsor shall discontinue the investigation as soon as possible, and in no event later than 5 working days after making the determination that the investigation should be discontinued. Upon request, FDA will confer with a sponsor on the need to discontinue an investigation.

21 CFR § 812.46 Monitoring investigations (medical devices)

(a) *Securing compliance.* A sponsor who discovers that an investigator is not complying with the signed agreement, the investigational plan, the requirements of this part or other applicable FDA regulations, or any conditions of approval imposed by the reviewing IRB or FDA shall promptly either secure compliance, or discontinue shipments of the device to the investigator and terminate the investigator's participation in the investigation. A sponsor shall also require such an investigator to dispose of or return the device, unless this action would jeopardize the rights, safety, or welfare of a subject.

(b) *Unanticipated adverse device effects.* (1) A sponsor shall immediately conduct an evaluation of any unanticipated adverse device effect. (2) A sponsor who determines that an unanticipated adverse device effect presents an unreasonable risk to subjects shall terminate all investigations or parts of investigations presenting that risk as soon as possible. Termination shall occur not later than 5 working days after the sponsor makes this determination and not later than 15 working days after the sponsor first received notice of the effect.

(c) *Resumption of terminated studies.* If the device is a significant risk device, a sponsor may not resume a terminated investigation without IRB and FDA approval. If the device is not a significant risk device, a sponsor may not resume a terminated investigation without IRB approval and, if the investigation was terminated under paragraph (b)(2) of this section, FDA approval.

21 CFR § 312.57 Recordkeeping and record retention (investigational drugs)

(a) A sponsor shall maintain adequate records showing the receipt, shipment, or other disposition of the investigational drug. These records are required to include, as appropriate, the name of the investigator to whom the drug is shipped, and the date, quantity, and batch or code mark of each such shipment.

(b) A sponsor shall maintain complete and accurate records showing any financial interest in §54.4(a)(3)(i), (a)(3)(ii), (a)(3)(iii), and (a)(3)(iv) of this chapter paid to clinical investigators by the sponsor of the covered study. A sponsor shall also maintain complete and accurate records concerning all other financial interests of investigators subject to part 54 of this chapter.

(c) A sponsor shall retain the records and reports required by this part for 2 years after a marketing application is approved for the drug; or, if an application is not approved for the drug, until 2 years after shipment and delivery of the drug for investigational use is discontinued and FDA has been so notified.

(d) A sponsor shall retain reserve samples of any test article and reference standard identified in, and used in any of the bioequivalence or bioavailability studies described in §320.38 or §320.63 of this chapter, and release the reserve samples to FDA upon request, in accordance with, and for the period specified in, §320.38.

21 CFR § 312.58 Inspection of sponsor's records and reports (investigational drugs)

(a) *FDA inspection.* A sponsor shall upon request from any properly authorized officer or employee of the Food and Drug Administration, at reasonable times, permit such officer or employee to have access to and copy and verify any records and reports relating to a clinical investigation conducted under this part. Upon written request by FDA, the sponsor shall submit the records or reports (or copies of them) to FDA. The sponsor shall discontinue shipments of the drug to any investigator who has failed to maintain or make available records or reports of the investigation as required by this part.

(b) *Controlled substances.* If any investigational new drug is a substance listed in any schedule of the Controlled Substances Act, records concerning shipment, delivery, receipt, and disposition of the drug, which are required to be kept under this part or other applicable parts of this chapter shall, upon the request of a properly authorized employee of the Drug Enforcement Administration of the U.S. Department of Justice, be made available by the investigator or sponsor, to whom the request is made, for inspection and copying. In addition, the sponsor shall assure that adequate precautions are taken, including storage of the investigational drug in a securely locked, substantially constructed cabinet, or other securely locked, substantially constructed enclosure, access to which is limited, to prevent theft or diversion of the substance into illegal channels of distribution.

21 CFR § 312.59 Disposition of unused supply of investigational drug (investigational drugs)
The sponsor shall assure the return of all unused supplies of the investigational drug from each

individual investigator whose participation in the investigation is discontinued or terminated. The sponsor may authorize alternative disposition of unused supplies of the investigational drug provided this alternative disposition does not expose humans to risks from the drug. The sponsor shall maintain written records of any disposition of the drug in accordance with §312.57.

Regulations Regarding Financial Disclosure by Clinical Investigators

21 CFR § 54.4 Certificate and disclosure requirements

(a)   The applicant that relies in whole or in part on clinical studies shall submit, for each clinical investigator who participated in a covered clinical study, either a certification described in paragraph (a)(1) of this section or a disclosure statement described in paragraph (a)(3) of this section.

(1) Certification: The applicant covered by this section shall submit for all clinical investigators [as defined in §54.2(d)], to whom the certification applies, a completed Form FDA 3454 attesting to the absence of financial interests and arrangements described in paragraph (a)(3) of this section. The form shall be dated and signed by the chief financial officer or other responsible corporate representative.

(2) If the certification covers less than all covered clinical data in the application, the applicant shall include in the certification a list of the studies covered by this certification.

(3) Disclosure Statement: For any clinical investigator defined in §54.2(d)for whom the applicant does not submit the certification described in paragraph (a)(1) of this section, the applicant shall submit a completed Form FDA 3455 disclosing completely and accurately the following:

(i) any financial arrangement entered into between the sponsor of the covered study and the clinical investigator involved in the conduct of a covered clinical trial, whereby the value of the compensation to the clinical investigator for conducting the study could be influenced by the outcome of the study;
(ii) any significant payments of other sorts from the sponsor of the covered study, such as a grant to fund ongoing research, compensation in the form of equipment, retainer for ongoing consultation, or honoraria;
(iii) any proprietary interest in the tested product held by any clinical investigator involved in a study;
(iv) any significant equity interest in the sponsor of the covered study held by any clinical investigator involved in any clinical study; and
(v) any steps taken to minimize the potential for bias resulting from any of the disclosed arrangements, interests, or payments.

(b)   The clinical investigator shall provide to the sponsor of the covered study sufficient accurate financial information to allow the sponsor to submit complete and accurate financial certification or disclosure statements as required in paragraph (a) of this section. The investigator shall promptly update this information if any relevant changes occur in the course of the investigation or for 1 year following completion of the study.

(c)   Refusal to file application. FDA may refuse to file any marketing application described in paragraph (a) of this section that does not contain the information required by this section or a certification by the applicant that the applicant has acted with due diligence to obtain the information but was unable to do so and stating the reason.

Friday
May 9, 1997

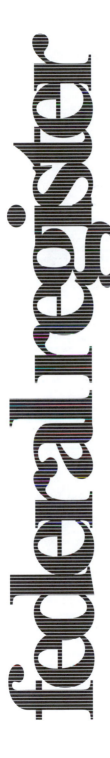

Part II

Department of Health and Human Services

Food and Drug Administration

International Conference on Harmonisation; Good Clinical Practice: Consolidated Guideline; Notice of Availability

DEPARTMENT OF HEALTH AND HUMAN SERVICES

Food and Drug Administration

[Docket No. 95D±0219]

International Conference on Harmonisation; Good Clinical Practice: Consolidated Guideline; Availability

AGENCY: Food and Drug Administration, HHS.

ACTION: Notice.

SUMMARY: The Food and Drug Administration (FDA) is publishing a guideline entitled "Good Clinical Practice: Consolidated Guideline." The guideline was prepared under the auspices of the International Conference on Harmonisation of Technical Requirements for Registration of Pharmaceuticals for Human Use (ICH). The guideline is intended to define "Good Clinical Practice" and to provide a unified standard for designing, conducting, recording, and reporting trials that involve the participation of human subjects. The guideline also describes the minimum information that should be included in an Investigator's Brochure (IB) and provides a suggested format. In addition, the guideline describes the essential documents that individually and collectively permit evaluation of the conduct of a clinical study and the quality of the data produced.

DATES: Effective May 9, 1997. Written comments may be submitted at any time.

ADDRESSES: Submit written requests for single copies of "Good Clinical Practice: Consolidated Guideline" to the Drug Information Branch (HFD±210), Center for Drug Evaluation and Research, Food and Drug Administration, 5600 Fishers Lane, Rockville, MD 20857, 301±827±□ 4573. Send two self-addressed adhesive labels to assist that office in processing your requests. Submit written comments on the guideline to the Dockets Management Branch (HFA±305), Food and Drug Administration, 12420 Parklawn Dr., rm. 1±23, Rockville, MD 20857. Two copies of any comments are to be submitted, except that individuals may submit one copy. The "Good Clinical Practice: Consolidated Guideline" and received comments are available for public examination in the Dockets Management Branch (address above) between 9 a.m. and 4 p.m., Monday through Friday.

FOR FURTHER INFORMATION CONTACT:
Regarding the guideline: Bette L. Barton, Center for Drug Evaluation and Research (HFD±344), Food and Drug Administration, 7500 Standish Pl., Rockville, MD 20855, 301±594±□ 1032.
Regarding ICH: Janet J. Showalter, Office of Health Affairs (HFY±20), Food and Drug Administration, 5600 Fishers Lane, Rockville, MD 20857, 301±827±0864.

SUPPLEMENTARY INFORMATION: In recent years, many important initiatives have been undertaken by regulatory authorities and industry associations to promote international harmonization of regulatory requirements. FDA has participated in many meetings designed to enhance harmonization and is committed to seeking scientifically based harmonized technical procedures for pharmaceutical development. One of the goals of harmonization is to identify and then reduce differences in technical requirements for drug development among regulatory agencies.

ICH was organized to provide an opportunity for tripartite harmonization initiatives to be developed with input from both regulatory and industry representatives. FDA also seeks input from consumer representatives and others. ICH is concerned with harmonization of technical requirements for the registration of pharmaceutical products among three regions: The European Union, Japan, and the United States. The six ICH sponsors are the European Commission, the European Federation of Pharmaceutical Industries Associations, the Japanese Ministry of Health and Welfare, the Japanese Pharmaceutical Manufacturers Association, the Centers for Drug Research and Research and Biologics Evaluation and Research, FDA, and the Pharmaceutical Research and Manufacturers of America. The ICH Secretariat, which coordinates the preparation of documentation, is provided by the International Federation of Pharmaceutical Manufacturers Associations (IFPMA).

The ICH Steering Committee includes representatives from each of the ICH sponsors and the IFPMA, as well as observers from the World Health Organization, the Canadian Health Protection Branch, and the European Free Trade Area.

In the **Federal Register** of August 17, 1995 (60 FR 42948), FDA published a draft tripartite guideline entitled "Good Clinical Practice." In the **Federal Register** of August 9, 1994, FDA published draft tripartite guidelines entitled "Guideline for the Investigator's Brochure" (59 FR 40772) and "Guideline for Essential Documents for the Conduct of a Clinical Study" (59 FR 40774). The notices gave interested persons an opportunity to submit comments.

After consideration of the comments received and revisions to the guidelines, the three guidelines were consolidated into one guideline on good clinical practice. The consolidated guideline was submitted to the ICH Steering Committee and endorsed by the three participating regulatory agencies at the ICH meeting held on April 30, 1996.

The guideline defines "Good Clinical Practice" and provides a unified standard for designing, conducting, recording, and reporting trials that involve the participation of human subjects. Compliance with Good Clinical Practice provides public assurance that the rights, well-being, and confidentiality of trial subjects are protected and that trial data are credible. The guideline should be followed when generating clinical data that are intended to be submitted to regulatory authorities. The principles established in this guideline should also be applied to other investigations that involve therapeutic intervention in, or observation of, human subjects.

The guideline also describes the minimum information that should be included in an IB, such as information on the drug's physical, chemical, and pharmaceutical properties, and its effect in humans; a suggested format for the IB is also provided. The guideline also describes the purpose of essential documents in a clinical study and explains whether the documents should be filed in the investigator's files or the sponsor's files.

This guideline represents the agency's current thinking on good clinical practices. It does not create or confer any rights for or on any person and does not operate to bind FDA or the public. An alternative approach may be used if such approach satisfies the requirements of the applicable statutes, regulations, or both.

As with all of FDA's guidelines, the public is encouraged to submit written comments with new data or other new information pertinent to this guideline. The comments in the docket will be periodically reviewed, and, where appropriate, the guideline will be amended. The public will be notified of any such amendments through a notice in the **Federal Register**.

Interested persons may, at any time, submit to the Dockets Management Branch (address above) written comments on the guideline. Two copies of any comments are to be submitted, except that individuals may submit one copy. Comments are to be identified with the docket number found in brackets in the heading of this document. A copy of the guideline and received comments may be seen in the office above between 9 a.m. and 4 p.m., Monday through Friday.

An electronic version of this guideline is available via Internet. Type http://www.fda.gov/cder and go to the "Regulatory Guidance" section.

The text of the guideline follows:

Good Clinical Practice: Consolidated Guideline

Introduction

Good clinical practice (GCP) is an international ethical and scientific quality standard for designing, conducting, recording, and reporting trials that involve the participation of human subjects. Compliance with this standard provides public assurance that the rights, safety, and well-being of trial subjects are protected, consistent with the principles that have their origin in the Declaration of Helsinki, and that clinical trial data are credible.

The objective of this ICH GCP Guideline is to provide a unified standard for the European Union (EU), Japan, and the United States to facilitate the mutual acceptance of clinical data by the regulatory authorities in these jurisdictions.

The guideline was developed with consideration of the current good clinical practices of the European Union, Japan, and the United States, as well as those of Australia, Canada, the Nordic countries, and the World Health Organization (WHO).

This guideline should be followed when generating clinical trial data that are intended to be submitted to regulatory authorities.

The principles established in this guideline may also be applied to other clinical investigations that may have an impact on the safety and well-being of human subjects.

1. Glossary

1.1 Adverse Drug Reaction (ADR)

In the preapproval clinical experience with a new medicinal product or its new usages, particularly as the therapeutic dose(s) may not be established, all noxious and unintended responses to a medicinal product related to any dose should be considered adverse drug reactions. The phrase "responses to a medicinal product" means that a causal relationship between a medicinal product and an adverse event is at least a reasonable possibility, i.e., the relationship cannot be ruled out.

Regarding marketed medicinal products: A response to a drug that is noxious and unintended and that occurs at doses normally used in man for prophylaxis, diagnosis, or therapy of diseases or for modification of physiological function (see the ICH Guideline for Clinical Safety Data Management: Definitions and Standards for Expedited Reporting).

1.2 Adverse Event (AE)

An AE is any untoward medical occurrence in a patient or clinical investigation subject administered a pharmaceutical product and that does not necessarily have a causal relationship with this treatment. An AE can therefore be any unfavorable and unintended sign (including an abnormal laboratory finding), symptom, or disease temporally associated with the use of a medicinal (investigational) product, whether or not related to the medicinal (investigational) product (see the ICH Guideline for Clinical Safety Data Management: Definitions and Standards for Expedited Reporting).

1.3 Amendment (to the protocol)

See Protocol Amendment.

1.4 Applicable Regulatory Requirement(s)

Any law(s) and regulation(s) addressing the conduct of clinical trials of investigational products of the jurisdiction where a trial is conducted.

1.5 Approval (in relation to Institutional Review Boards (IRB's))

The affirmative decision of the IRB that the clinical trial has been reviewed and may be conducted at the institution site within the constraints set forth by the IRB, the institution, good clinical practice (GCP), and the applicable regulatory requirements.

1.6 Audit

A systematic and independent examination of trial-related activities and documents to determine whether the evaluated trial-related activities were conducted, and the data were recorded, analyzed, and accurately reported according to the protocol, sponsor's standard operating procedures (SOP's), good clinical practice (GCP), and the applicable regulatory requirement(s).

1.7 *Audit Certificate*

A declaration of confirmation by the auditor that an audit has taken place.

1.8 *Audit Report*

A written evaluation by the sponsor's auditor of the results of the audit.

1.9 *Audit Trail*

Documentation that allows reconstruction of the course of events.

1.10 *Blinding/Masking*

A procedure in which one or more parties to the trial are kept unaware of the treatment assignment(s). Single blinding usually refers to the subject(s) being unaware, and double blinding usually refers to the subject(s), investigator(s), monitor, and, in some cases, data analyst(s) being unaware of the treatment assignment(s).

1.11 *Case Report Form (CRF)*

A printed, optical, or electronic document designed to record all of the protocol-required information to be reported to the sponsor on each trial subject.

1.12 *Clinical Trial/Study*

Any investigation in human subjects intended to discover or verify the clinical, pharmacological, and/or other pharmacodynamic effects of an investigational product(s), and/or to identify any adverse reactions to an investigational product(s), and/or to study absorption, distribution, metabolism, and excretion of an investigational product(s) with the object of ascertaining its safety and/or efficacy. The terms clinical trial and clinical study are synonymous.

1.13 *Clinical Trial/Study Report*

A written description of a trial/study of any therapeutic, prophylactic, or diagnostic agent conducted in human subjects, in which the clinical and statistical description, presentations, and analyses are fully integrated into a single report (see the ICH Guideline for Structure and Content of Clinical Study Reports).

1.14 *Comparator (Product)*

An investigational or marketed product (i.e., active control), or placebo, used as a reference in a clinical trial.

1.15 *Compliance (in relation to trials)*

Adherence to all the trial-related requirements, good clinical practice (GCP) requirements, and the applicable regulatory requirements.

1.16 *Confidentiality*

Prevention of disclosure, to other than authorized individuals, of a sponsor's proprietary information or of a subject's identity.

1.17 *Contract*

A written, dated, and signed agreement between two or more involved parties that sets out any arrangements on delegation and distribution of tasks and obligations and, if appropriate, on financial matters. The protocol may serve as the basis of a contract.

1.18 *Coordinating Committee*

A committee that a sponsor may organize to coordinate the conduct of a multicenter trial.

1.19 *Coordinating Investigator*

An investigator assigned the responsibility for the coordination of investigators at different centers participating in a multicenter trial.

1.20 *Contract Research Organization (CRO)*

A person or an organization (commercial, academic, or other) contracted by the sponsor to perform one or more of a sponsor's trial-related duties and functions.

1.21 *Direct Access*

Permission to examine, analyze, verify, and reproduce any records and reports that are important to evaluation of a clinical trial. Any party (e.g., domestic and foreign regulatory authorities, sponsors, monitors, and auditors) with direct access should take all reasonable precautions within the constraints of the applicable regulatory requirement(s) to maintain the confidentiality of subjects' identities and sponsor's proprietary information.

1.22 *Documentation*

All records, in any form (including, but not limited to, written, electronic, magnetic, and optical records; and scans, x-rays, and electrocardiograms) that describe or record the methods, conduct, and/or results of a trial, the factors affecting a trial, and the actions taken.

1.23 *Essential Documents*

Documents that individually and collectively permit evaluation of the conduct of a study and the quality of the data produced (see 8. "Essential Documents for the Conduct of a Clinical Trial").

1.24 *Good Clinical Practice (GCP)*

A standard for the design, conduct, performance, monitoring, auditing, recording, analyses, and reporting of clinical trials that provides assurance that the data and reported results are credible and accurate, and that the rights, integrity, and confidentiality of trial subjects are protected.

1.25 *Independent Data Monitoring Committee (IDMC) (Data and Safety Monitoring Board, Monitoring Committee, Data Monitoring Committee)*

An independent data monitoring committee that may be established by the sponsor to assess at intervals the progress of a clinical trial, the safety data, and the critical efficacy endpoints, and to recommend to the sponsor whether to continue, modify, or stop a trial.

1.26 *Impartial Witness*

A person, who is independent of the trial, who cannot be unfairly influenced by people involved with the trial, who attends the informed consent process if the subject or the subject's legally acceptable representative cannot read, and who reads the informed consent form and any other written information supplied to the subject.

1.27 *Independent Ethics Committee (IEC)*

An independent body (a review board or a committee, institutional, regional, national, or supranational), constituted of medical/scientific professionals and nonmedical/nonscientific members, whose responsibility it is to ensure the protection of the rights, safety, and well-being of human subjects involved in a trial and to provide public assurance of that protection, by, among other things, reviewing and approving/providing favorable opinion on the trial protocol, the

suitability of the investigator(s), facilities, and the methods and material to be used in obtaining and documenting informed consent of the trial subjects.

The legal status, composition, function, operations, and regulatory requirements pertaining to Independent Ethics Committees may differ among countries, but should allow the Independent Ethics Committee to act in agreement with GCP as described in this guideline.

1.28 *Informed Consent*

A process by which a subject voluntarily confirms his or her willingness to participate in a particular trial, after having been informed of all aspects of the trial that are relevant to the subject's decision to participate. Informed consent is documented by means of a written, signed, and dated informed consent form.

1.29 *Inspection*

The act by a regulatory authority(ies) of conducting an official review of documents, facilities, records, and any other resources that are deemed by the authority(ies) to be related to the clinical trial and that may be located at the site of the trial, at the sponsor's and/or contract research organization's (CRO's) facilities, or at other establishments deemed appropriate by the regulatory authority(ies).

1.30 *Institution (medical)*

Any public or private entity or agency or medical or dental facility where clinical trials are conducted.

1.31 *Institutional Review Board (IRB)*

An independent body constituted of medical, scientific, and nonscientific members, whose responsibility it is to ensure the protection of the rights, safety, and well-being of human subjects involved in a trial by, among other things, reviewing, approving, and providing continuing review of trials, of protocols and amendments, and of the methods and material to be used in obtaining and documenting informed consent of the trial subjects.

1.32 *Interim Clinical Trial/Study Report*

A report of intermediate results and their evaluation based on analyses performed during the course of a trial.

1.33 *Investigational Product*

A pharmaceutical form of an active ingredient or placebo being tested or used as a reference in a clinical trial, including a product with a marketing authorization when used or assembled (formulated or packaged) in a way different from the approved form, or when used for an unapproved indication, or when used to gain further information about an approved use.

1.34 *Investigator*

A person responsible for the conduct of the clinical trial at a trial site. If a trial is conducted by a team of individuals at a trial site, the investigator is the responsible leader of the team and may be called the principal investigator. See also Subinvestigator.

1.35 *Investigator/Institution*

An expression meaning "the investigator and/or institution, where required by the applicable regulatory requirements."

1.36 *Investigator's Brochure*

A compilation of the clinical and nonclinical data on the investigational product(s) that is relevant to the study of the investigational product(s) in human subjects (see 7. "Investigator's Brochure").

1.37 *Legally Acceptable Representative*
An individual or juridical or other body authorized under applicable law to consent, on behalf of a prospective subject, to the subject's participation in the clinical trial.

1.38 *Monitoring*
The act of overseeing the progress of a clinical trial, and of ensuring that it is conducted, recorded, and reported in accordance with the protocol, standard operating procedures (SOP's), GCP, and the applicable regulatory requirement(s).

1.39 *Monitoring Report*
A written report from the monitor to the sponsor after each site visit and/or other trial-related communication according to the sponsor's SOP's.

1.40 *Multicenter Trial*
A clinical trial conducted according to a single protocol but at more than one site, and, therefore, carried out by more than one investigator.

1.41 *Nonclinical Study*
Biomedical studies not performed on human subjects.

1.42 *Opinion (in relation to Independent Ethics Committee)*
The judgment and/or the advice provided by an Independent Ethics Committee (IEC).

1.43 *Original Medical Record*
See Source Documents.

1.44 *Protocol*
A document that describes the objective(s), design, methodology, statistical considerations, and organization of a trial. The protocol usually also gives the background and rationale for the trial, but these could be provided in other protocol referenced documents. Throughout the ICH GCP Guideline, the term protocol refers to protocol and protocol amendments.

1.45 *Protocol Amendment*
A written description of a change(s) to or formal clarification of a protocol.

1.46 *Quality Assurance (QA)*
All those planned and systematic actions that are established to ensure that the trial is performed and the data are generated, documented (recorded), and reported in compliance with GCP and the applicable regulatory requirement(s).

1.47 *Quality Control (QC)*
The operational techniques and activities undertaken within the quality assurance system to verify that the requirements for quality of the trial-related activities have been fulfilled.

1.48 *Randomization*
The process of assigning trial subjects to treatment or control groups using an element of chance to determine the assignments in order to reduce bias.

1.49 *Regulatory Authorities*
Bodies having the power to regulate. In the ICH GCP guideline, the expression "Regulatory Authorities" includes the authorities that review submitted clinical data and those that conduct inspections (see 1.29). These bodies are sometimes referred to as competent authorities.

1.50 *Serious Adverse Event (SAE) or Serious Adverse Drug Reaction (Serious ADR)*
Any untoward medical occurrence that at any dose:

- Results in death,
- Is life-threatening,
- Requires inpatient hospitalization or prolongation of existing hospitalization,
- Results in persistent or significant disability/incapacity,
or
- Is a congenital anomaly/birth defect.
(See the ICH Guideline for Clinical Safety Data Management: Definitions and Standards for Expedited Reporting.)

1.51 *Source Data*
All information in original records and certified copies of original records of clinical findings, observations, or other activities in a clinical trial necessary for the reconstruction and evaluation of the trial. Source data are contained in source documents (original records or certified copies).

1.52 *Source Documents*
Original documents, data, and records (e.g., hospital records, clinical and office charts, laboratory notes, memoranda, subjects' diaries or evaluation checklists, pharmacy dispensing records, recorded data from automated instruments, copies or transcriptions certified after verification as being accurate and complete, microfiches, photographic negatives, microfilm or magnetic media, x-rays, subject files, and records kept at the pharmacy, at the laboratories, and at medico-technical departments involved in the clinical trial).

1.53 *Sponsor*
An individual, company, institution, or organization that takes responsibility for the initiation, management, and/or financing of a clinical trial.

1.54 *Sponsor-Investigator*
An individual who both initiates and conducts, alone or with others, a clinical trial, and under whose immediate direction the investigational product is administered to, dispensed to, or used by a subject. The term does not include any person other than an individual (e.g., it does not include a corporation or an agency). The obligations of a sponsor-investigator include both those of a sponsor and those of an investigator.

1.55 *Standard Operating Procedures (SOP's)*
Detailed, written instructions to achieve uniformity of the performance of a specific function.

1.56 *Subinvestigator*
Any individual member of the clinical trial team designated and supervised by the investigator at a trial site to perform critical trial-related procedures and/or to make important trial-related decisions (e.g., associates, residents, research fellows). See also Investigator.

1.57 *Subject/Trial Subject*
An individual who participates in a clinical trial, either as a recipient of the investigational product(s) or as a control.

1.58 *Subject Identification Code*
A unique identifier assigned by the investigator to each trial subject to protect the subject's identity and used in lieu of the subject's name when the investigator reports adverse events and/or other trial-related data.

1.59 *Trial Site*
The location(s) where trial-related activities are actually conducted.

1.60 *Unexpected Adverse Drug Reaction*

An adverse reaction, the nature or severity of which is not consistent with the applicable product information (e.g., Investigator's Brochure for an unapproved investigational product or package insert/summary of product characteristics for an approved product). (See the ICH Guideline for Clinical Safety Data Management: Definitions and Standards for Expedited Reporting.)

1.61 *Vulnerable Subjects*
Individuals whose willingness to volunteer in a clinical trial may be unduly influenced by the expectation, whether justified or not, of benefits associated with participation, or of a retaliatory response from senior members of a hierarchy in case of refusal to participate. Examples are members of a group with a hierarchical structure, such as medical, pharmacy, dental, and nursing students, subordinate hospital and laboratory personnel, employees of the pharmaceutical industry, members of the armed forces, and persons kept in detention. Other vulnerable subjects include patients with incurable diseases, persons in nursing homes, unemployed or impoverished persons, patients in emergency situations, ethnic minority groups, homeless persons, nomads, refugees, minors, and those incapable of giving consent.

1.62 *Well-being (of the trial subjects)*
The physical and mental integrity of the subjects participating in a clinical trial.

2. *The Principles of ICH GCP*

2.1 Clinical trials should be conducted in accordance with the ethical principles that have their origin in the Declaration of Helsinki, and that are consistent with GCP and the applicable regulatory requirement(s).

2.2 Before a trial is initiated, foreseeable risks and inconveniences should be weighed against the anticipated benefit for the individual trial subject and society. A trial should be initiated and continued only if the anticipated benefits justify the risks.

2.3 The rights, safety, and well-being of the trial subjects are the most important considerations and should prevail over interests of science and society.

2.4 The available nonclinical and clinical information on an investigational product should be adequate to support the proposed clinical trial.

2.5 Clinical trials should be scientifically sound, and described in a clear, detailed protocol.

2.6 A trial should be conducted in compliance with the protocol that has received prior institutional review board (IRB)/independent ethics committee (IEC) approval/favorable opinion.

2.7 The medical care given to, and medical decisions made on behalf of, subjects should always be the responsibility of a qualified physician or, when appropriate, of a qualified dentist.

2.8 Each individual involved in conducting a trial should be qualified by education, training, and experience to perform his or her respective task(s).

2.9 Freely given informed consent should be obtained from every subject prior to clinical trial participation.

2.10 All clinical trial information should be recorded, handled, and stored in a way that allows its accurate reporting, interpretation, and verification.

2.11 The confidentiality of records that could identify subjects should be protected, respecting the privacy and confidentiality rules in accordance with the applicable regulatory requirement(s).

2.12 Investigational products should be manufactured, handled, and stored in accordance with applicable good manufacturing practice (GMP). They should be used in accordance with the approved protocol.

2.13 Systems with procedures that assure the quality of every aspect of the trial should be implemented.

3. *Institutional Review Board/Independent Ethics Committee (IRB/IEC)*

3.1 *Responsibilities*

3.1.1 An IRB/IEC should safeguard the rights, safety, and well-being of all trial subjects. Special attention should be paid to trials that may include vulnerable subjects.

3.1.2 The IRB/IEC should obtain the following documents:

Trial protocol(s)/amendment(s), written informed consent form(s) and consent form updates that the investigator proposes for use in the trial, subject recruitment procedures (e.g., advertisements), written information to be provided to subjects, Investigator's Brochure (IB), available safety information, information about payments and compensation available to subjects, the investigator's current curriculum vitae and/or other documentation evidencing qualifications, and any other documents that the IRB/IEC may require to fulfill its responsibilities.

The IRB/IEC should review a proposed clinical trial within a reasonable time and document its views in writing, clearly identifying the trial, the documents reviewed, and the dates for the following:

- Approval/favorable opinion;
- Modifications required prior to its approval/favorable opinion;
- Disapproval/negative opinion; and
- Termination/suspension of any prior approval/favorable opinion.

3.1.3 The IRB/IEC should consider the qualifications of the investigator for the proposed trial, as documented by a current curriculum vitae and/or by any other relevant documentation the IRB/IEC requests.

3.1.4 The IRB/IEC should conduct continuing review of each ongoing trial at intervals appropriate to the degree of risk to human subjects, but at least once per year.

3.1.5 The IRB/IEC may request more information than is outlined in paragraph 4.8.10 be given to subjects when, in the judgment of the IRB/IEC, the additional information would add meaningfully to the protection of the rights, safety, and/or well-being of the subjects.

3.1.6 When a nontherapeutic trial is to be carried out with the consent of the subject's legally acceptable representative (see 4.8.12, 4.8.14), the IRB/IEC should determine that the proposed protocol and/or other document(s) adequately addresses relevant ethical concerns and meets applicable regulatory requirements for such trials.

3.1.7 Where the protocol indicates that prior consent of the trial subject or the subject's legally acceptable representative is not possible (see 4.8.15), the IRB/IEC should determine that the proposed protocol and/or other document(s) adequately addresses relevant ethical concerns and meets applicable regulatory requirements for such trials (i.e., in emergency situations).

3.1.8 The IRB/IEC should review both the amount and method of payment to subjects to assure that neither presents problems of coercion or undue influence on the trial subjects. Payments to a subject should be prorated and not wholly contingent on completion of the trial by the subject.

3.1.9 The IRB/IEC should ensure that information regarding payment to subjects, including the methods, amounts, and schedule of payment to trial subjects, is set forth in the written informed consent form and any other written information to be provided to subjects. The way payment will be prorated should be specified.

3.2 *Composition, Functions, and Operations*

3.2.1 The IRB/IEC should consist of a reasonable number of members, who collectively have the qualifications and experience to review and evaluate the science, medical aspects, and ethics of the proposed trial. It is recommended that the IRB/IEC should include:

(a) At least five members.

(b) At least one member whose primary area of interest is in a nonscientific area.

(c) At least one member who is independent of the institution/trial site.

Only those IRB/IEC members who are independent of the investigator and the sponsor of the trial should vote/provide opinion on a trial-related matter.

A list of IRB/IEC members and their qualifications should be maintained.

3.2.2 The IRB/IEC should perform its functions according to written operating procedures, should maintain written records of its activities and minutes of its meetings, and should comply with GCP and with the applicable regulatory requirement(s).

3.2.3 An IRB/IEC should make its decisions at announced meetings at which at least a quorum, as stipulated in its written operating procedures, is present.

3.2.4 Only members who participate in the IRB/IEC review and discussion should vote/provide their opinion and/or advise.

3.2.5 The investigator may provide information on any aspect of the trial, but should not participate in the deliberations of the IRB/IEC or in the vote/opinion of the IRB/IEC.

3.2.6 An IRB/IEC may invite nonmembers with expertise in special areas for assistance.

3.3 *Procedures*

The IRB/IEC should establish, document in writing, and follow its procedures, which should include:

3.3.1 Determining its composition (names and qualifications of the members) and the authority under which it is established.

3.3.2 Scheduling, notifying its members of, and conducting its meetings.

3.3.3 Conducting initial and continuing review of trials.

3.3.4 Determining the frequency of continuing review, as appropriate.

3.3.5 Providing, according to the applicable regulatory requirements, expedited review and approval/favorable opinion of minor change(s) in ongoing trials that have the approval/favorable opinion of the IRB/IEC.

3.3.6 Specifying that no subject should be admitted to a trial before the IRB/IEC issues its written approval/favorable opinion of the trial.

3.3.7 Specifying that no deviations from, or changes of, the protocol should be initiated without prior written IRB/IEC approval/favorable opinion of an appropriate amendment, except when necessary to eliminate immediate hazards to the subjects or when the change(s) involves only logistical or administrative aspects of the trial (e.g., change of monitor(s), telephone number(s)) (see 4.5.2).

3.3.8 Specifying that the investigator should promptly report to the IRB/IEC:

(a) Deviations from, or changes of, the protocol to eliminate immediate hazards to the trial subjects (see 3.3.7, 4.5.2, 4.5.4).

(b) Changes increasing the risk to subjects and/or affecting significantly the conduct of the trial (see 4.10.2).

(c) All adverse drug reactions (ADR's) that are both serious and unexpected.

(d) New information that may affect adversely the safety of the subjects or the conduct of the trial.

3.3.9 Ensuring that the IRB/IEC promptly notify in writing the investigator/institution concerning:

(a) Its trial-related decisions/opinions.

(b) The reasons for its decisions/opinions.

(c) Procedures for appeal of its decisions/opinions.

3.4 *Records*

The IRB/IEC should retain all relevant records (e.g., written procedures, membership lists, lists of occupations/affiliations of members, submitted documents, minutes of meetings, and correspondence) for a period of at least 3 years after completion of the trial and make them available upon request from the regulatory authority(ies).

The IRB/IEC may be asked by investigators, sponsors, or regulatory authorities to provide copies of its written procedures and membership lists.

4. *Investigator*

4.1 *Investigator's Qualifications and Agreements*

4.1.1 The investigator(s) should be qualified by education, training, and experience to assume responsibility for the proper conduct of the trial, should meet all the qualifications specified by the applicable regulatory requirement(s), and should provide evidence of such qualifications through up-to-date curriculum vitae and/or other relevant documentation requested by the sponsor, the IRB/IEC, and/or the regulatory authority(ies).

4.1.2 The investigator should be thoroughly familiar with the appropriate use of the investigational product(s), as described in the protocol, in the current Investigator's Brochure, in the product information, and in other information sources provided by the sponsor.

4.1.3 The investigator should be aware of, and should comply with, GCP and the applicable regulatory requirements.

4.1.4 The investigator/institution should permit monitoring and auditing by the sponsor, and inspection by the appropriate regulatory authority(ies).

4.1.5 The investigator should maintain a list of appropriately qualified persons to whom the investigator has delegated significant trial-related duties.

4.2 *Adequate Resources*

4.2.1 The investigator should be able to demonstrate (e.g., based on retrospective data) a potential for recruiting the required number of suitable subjects within the agreed recruitment period.

4.2.2 The investigator should have sufficient time to properly conduct and complete the trial within the agreed trial period.

4.2.3 The investigator should have available an adequate number of qualified staff and adequate facilities for the foreseen duration of the trial to conduct the trial properly and safely.

4.2.4 The investigator should ensure that all persons assisting with the trial are adequately informed about the protocol, the investigational product(s), and their trial-related duties and functions.

4.3 *Medical Care of Trial Subjects*

4.3.1 A qualified physician (or dentist, when appropriate), who is an investigator or a subinvestigator for the trial, should be responsible for all trial-related medical (or dental) decisions.

4.3.2 During and following a subject's participation in a trial, the investigator/institution should ensure that adequate medical care is provided to a subject for any adverse events, including clinically significant laboratory values, related to the trial. The investigator/institution should inform a subject when medical care is needed for intercurrent illness(es) of which the investigator becomes aware.

4.3.3 It is recommended that the investigator inform the subject's primary physician about the subject's participation in the trial if the subject has a primary physician and if the subject agrees to the primary physician being informed.

4.3.4 Although a subject is not obliged to give his/her reason(s) for withdrawing prematurely from a trial, the investigator should make a reasonable effort to ascertain the reason(s), while fully respecting the subject's rights.

4.4 *Communication with IRB/IEC*

4.4.1 Before initiating a trial, the investigator/institution should have written and dated approval/favorable opinion from the IRB/IEC for the trial protocol, written informed consent form, consent form updates, subject recruitment procedures (e.g., advertisements), and any other written information to be provided to subjects.

4.4.2 As part of the investigator's/institution's written application to the IRB/IEC, the investigator/institution should provide the IRB/IEC with a current copy of the Investigator's Brochure. If the Investigator's Brochure is updated during the trial, the investigator/institution should supply a copy of the updated Investigator's Brochure to the IRB/IEC.

4.4.3 During the trial the investigator/institution should provide to the IRB/IEC all documents subject to its review.

4.5 *Compliance with Protocol*

4.5.1 The investigator/institution should conduct the trial in compliance with the protocol agreed to by the sponsor and, if required, by the regulatory authority(ies), and which was given approval/favorable opinion

by the IRB/IEC. The investigator/institution and the sponsor should sign the protocol, or an alternative contract, to confirm their agreement.

4.5.2 The investigator should not implement any deviation from, or changes of, the protocol without agreement by the sponsor and prior review and documented approval/favorable opinion from the IRB/IEC of an amendment, except where necessary to eliminate an immediate hazard(s) to trial subjects, or when the change(s) involves only logistical or administrative aspects of the trial (e.g., change of monitor(s), change of telephone number(s)).

4.5.3 The investigator, or person designated by the investigator, should document and explain any deviation from the approved protocol.

4.5.4 The investigator may implement a deviation from, or a change in, the protocol to eliminate an immediate hazard(s) to trial subjects without prior IRB/IEC approval/favorable opinion. As soon as possible, the implemented deviation or change, the reasons for it, and, if appropriate, the proposed protocol amendment(s) should be submitted:

(a) To the IRB/IEC for review and approval/favorable opinion;

(b) To the sponsor for agreement; and, if required,

(c) To the regulatory authority(ies).

4.6 *Investigational Product(s)*

4.6.1 Responsibility for investigational product(s) accountability at the trial site(s) rests with the investigator/institution.

4.6.2 Where allowed/required, the investigator/institution may/should assign some or all of the investigator's/institution's duties for investigational product(s) accountability at the trial site(s) to an appropriate pharmacist or another appropriate individual who is under the supervision of the investigator/institution.

4.6.3 The investigator/institution and/or a pharmacist or other appropriate individual, who is designated by the investigator/institution, should maintain records of the product's delivery to the trial site, the inventory at the site, the use by each subject, and the return to the sponsor or alternative disposition of unused product(s). These records should include dates, quantities, batch/serial numbers, expiration dates (if applicable), and the unique code numbers assigned to the investigational product(s) and trial subjects. Investigators should maintain records that document adequately that the subjects were provided the doses specified by the protocol and reconcile all investigational product(s) received from the sponsor.

4.6.4 The investigational product(s) should be stored as specified by the sponsor (see 5.13.2 and 5.14.3) and in accordance with applicable regulatory requirement(s).

4.6.5 The investigator should ensure that the investigational product(s) are used only in accordance with the approved protocol.

4.6.6 The investigator, or a person designated by the investigator/institution, should explain the correct use of the investigational product(s) to each subject and should check, at intervals appropriate for the trial, that each subject is following the instructions properly.

4.7 *Randomization Procedures and Unblinding*

The investigator should follow the trial's randomization procedures, if any, and should ensure that the code is broken only in accordance with the protocol. If the trial is blinded, the investigator should promptly document and explain to the sponsor any premature unblinding (e.g., accidental unblinding, unblinding due to a serious adverse event) of the investigational product(s).

4.8 *Informed Consent of Trial Subjects*

4.8.1 In obtaining and documenting informed consent, the investigator should comply with the applicable regulatory requirement(s), and should adhere to GCP and to the ethical principles that have their origin in the Declaration of Helsinki. Prior to the beginning of the trial, the investigator should have the IRB/IEC's written approval/favorable opinion of the written informed consent form and any other written information to be provided to subjects.

4.8.2 The written informed consent form and any other written information to be provided to subjects should be revised whenever important new information becomes available that may be relevant to the subject's consent. Any revised written informed consent form, and written information should receive the IRB/IEC's approval/favorable opinion in advance of use. The subject or the subject's legally acceptable representative should be informed in a timely manner if new information becomes available that may be relevant to the subject's willingness to continue participation in the trial. The communication of this information should be documented.

4.8.3 Neither the investigator, nor the trial staff, should coerce or unduly influence a subject to participate or to continue to participate in a trial.

4.8.4 None of the oral and written information concerning the trial, including the written informed consent form, should contain any language that causes the subject or the subject's legally acceptable representative to waive or to appear to waive any legal rights, or that releases or appears to release the investigator, the institution, the sponsor, or their agents from liability for negligence.

4.8.5 The investigator, or a person designated by the investigator, should fully inform the subject or, if the subject is unable to provide informed consent, the subject's legally acceptable representative, of all pertinent aspects of the trial including the written information given approval/favorable opinion by the IRB/IEC.

4.8.6 The language used in the oral and written information about the trial, including the written informed consent form, should be as nontechnical as practical and should be understandable to the subject or the subject's legally acceptable representative and the impartial witness, where applicable.

4.8.7 Before informed consent may be obtained, the investigator, or a person designated by the investigator, should provide the subject or the subject's legally acceptable representative ample time and opportunity to inquire about details of the trial and to decide whether or not to participate in the trial. All questions about the trial should be answered to the satisfaction of the subject or the subject's legally acceptable representative.

4.8.8 Prior to a subject's participation in the trial, the written informed consent form should be signed and personally dated by the subject or by the subject's legally acceptable representative, and by the person who conducted the informed consent discussion.

4.8.9 If a subject is unable to read or if a legally acceptable representative is unable to read, an impartial witness should be present during the entire informed consent discussion. After the written informed consent form and any other written information to be provided to subjects is read and explained to the subject or the subject's legally acceptable representative, and after the subject or the subject's legally acceptable representative has orally consented to the subject's participation in the trial, and, if capable of doing so, has signed and personally dated the informed consent form, the witness should sign and personally date the consent form. By signing the consent form, the witness attests that the information in the consent form and any other written information was accurately explained to, and apparently understood by, the subject or the subject's legally acceptable representative, and that informed consent was freely given by the subject or the subject's legally acceptable representative.

4.8.10 Both the informed consent discussion and the written informed consent form and any other written information to be provided to subjects should include explanations of the following:

(a) That the trial involves research.

(b) The purpose of the trial.

(c) The trial treatment(s) and the probability for random assignment to each treatment.

(d) The trial procedures to be followed, including all invasive procedures.

(e) The subject's responsibilities.

(f) Those aspects of the trial that are experimental.

(g) The reasonably foreseeable risks or inconveniences to the subject and, when applicable, to an embryo, fetus, or nursing infant.

(h) The reasonably expected benefits. When there is no intended clinical benefit to the subject, the subject should be made aware of this.

(i) The alternative procedure(s) or course(s) of treatment that may be available to the subject, and their important potential benefits and risks.

(j) The compensation and/or treatment available to the subject in the event of trial-related injury.

(k) The anticipated prorated payment, if any, to the subject for participating in the trial.

(l) The anticipated expenses, if any, to the subject for participating in the trial.

(m) That the subject's participation in the trial is voluntary and that the subject may refuse to participate or withdraw from the trial, at any time, without penalty or loss of benefits to which the subject is otherwise entitled.

(n) That the monitor(s), the auditor(s), the IRB/IEC, and the regulatory authority(ies) will be granted direct access to the subject's original medical records for verification of clinical trial procedures and/or data, without violating the confidentiality of the subject, to the extent permitted by the applicable laws and regulations and that, by signing a written informed consent form, the subject or the subject's legally acceptable representative is authorizing such access.

(o) That records identifying the subject will be kept confidential and, to the extent permitted by the applicable laws and/or regulations, will not be made publicly available. If the results of the trial are published, the subject's identity will remain confidential.

(p) That the subject or the subject's legally acceptable representative will be informed in a timely manner if information becomes available that may be relevant to the subject's willingness to continue participation in the trial.

(q) The person(s) to contact for further information regarding the trial and the rights of trial subjects, and whom to contact in the event of trial-related injury.

(r) The foreseeable circumstances and/or reasons under which the subject's participation in the trial may be terminated.

(s) The expected duration of the subject's participation in the trial.

(t) The approximate number of subjects involved in the trial.

4.8.11 Prior to participation in the trial, the subject or the subject's legally acceptable representative should receive a copy of the signed and dated written informed consent form and any other written information provided to the subjects. During a subject's participation in the trial, the subject or the subject's legally acceptable representative should receive a copy of the signed and dated consent form updates and a copy of any amendments to the written information provided to subjects.

4.8.12 When a clinical trial (therapeutic or nontherapeutic) includes subjects who can only be enrolled in the trial with the consent of the subject's legally acceptable representative (e.g., minors, or patients with severe dementia), the subject should be informed about the trial to the extent compatible with the subject's understanding and, if capable, the subject should assent, sign and personally date the written informed consent.

4.8.13 Except as described in 4.8.14, a nontherapeutic trial (i.e., a trial in which there is no anticipated direct clinical benefit to the subject) should be conducted in subjects who personally give consent and who sign and date the written informed consent form.

4.8.14 Nontherapeutic trials may be conducted in subjects with consent of a legally acceptable representative provided the following conditions are fulfilled:

(a) The objectives of the trial cannot be met by means of a trial in subjects who can give informed consent personally.

(b) The foreseeable risks to the subjects are low.

(c) The negative impact on the subject's well-being is minimized and low.

(d) The trial is not prohibited by law.

(e) The approval/favorable opinion of the IRB/IEC is expressly sought on the inclusion of such subjects, and the written approval/favorable opinion covers this aspect.

Such trials, unless an exception is justified, should be conducted in patients having a disease or condition for which the investigational product is intended. Subjects in these trials should be particularly closely monitored and should be withdrawn if they appear to be unduly distressed.

4.8.15 In emergency situations, when prior consent of the subject is not possible, the consent of the subject's legally acceptable representative, if present, should be requested. When prior consent of the subject is not possible, and the subject's legally acceptable representative is not available, enrollment of the subject should require measures described in the protocol and/or elsewhere, with documented approval/favorable opinion by the IRB/IEC, to protect the rights, safety, and well-being of the subject and to ensure compliance with applicable regulatory requirements. The subject or the subject's legally acceptable representative should be informed about the trial as soon as possible and consent to continue and other consent as appropriate (see 4.8.10) should be requested.

4.9 Records and Reports

4.9.1 The investigator should ensure the accuracy, completeness, legibility, and timeliness of the data reported to the sponsor in the CRF's and in all required reports.

4.9.2 Data reported on the CRF, which are derived from source documents, should be consistent with the source documents or the discrepancies should be explained.

4.9.3 Any change or correction to a CRF should be dated, initialed, and explained (if necessary) and should not obscure the original entry (i.e., an audit trail should be maintained); this applies to both written and electronic changes or corrections (see 5.18.4(n)). Sponsors should provide guidance to investigators and/or the investigators' designated representatives on making such corrections. Sponsors should have written procedures to assure that changes or corrections in CRF's made by sponsor's designated representatives are documented, are necessary, and are endorsed by the investigator. The investigator should retain records of the changes and corrections.

4.9.4 The investigator/institution should maintain the trial documents as specified in Essential Documents for the Conduct of a Clinical Trial (see 8.) and as required by the applicable regulatory requirement(s). The investigator/institution should take measures to prevent accidental or premature destruction of these documents.

4.9.5 Essential documents should be retained until at least 2 years after the last approval of a marketing application in an ICH region and until there are no pending or contemplated marketing applications in an ICH region or at least 2 years have elapsed since the formal discontinuation of clinical development of the investigational product. These documents should be retained for a longer period, however, if required by the applicable regulatory requirements or by an agreement with the sponsor. It is the responsibility of the sponsor to inform the investigator/institution as to when these documents no longer need to be retained (see 5.5.12).

238

4.9.6 The financial aspects of the trial should be documented in an agreement between the sponsor and the investigator/institution.

4.9.7 Upon request of the monitor, auditor, IRB/IEC, or regulatory authority, the investigator/institution should make available for direct access all requested trial-related records.

4.10 *Progress Reports*

4.10.1 Where required by the applicable regulatory requirements, the investigator should submit written summaries of the trial's status to the institution. The investigator/institution should submit written summaries of the status of the trial to the IRB/IEC annually, or more frequently, if requested by the IRB/IEC.

4.10.2 The investigator should promptly provide written reports to the sponsor, the IRB/IEC (see 3.3.8), and, where required by the applicable regulatory requirements, the institution on any changes significantly affecting the conduct of the trial, and/or increasing the risk to subjects.

4.11 *Safety Reporting*

4.11.1 All serious adverse events (SAE's) should be reported immediately to the sponsor except for those SAE's that the protocol or other document (e.g., Investigator's Brochure) identifies as not needing immediate reporting. The immediate reports should be followed promptly by detailed, written reports. The immediate and follow-up reports should identify subjects by unique code numbers assigned to the trial subjects rather than by the subjects' names, personal identification numbers, and/or addresses. The investigator should also comply with the applicable regulatory requirement(s) related to the reporting of unexpected serious adverse drug reactions to the regulatory authority(ies) and the IRB/IEC.

4.11.2 Adverse events and/or laboratory abnormalities identified in the protocol as critical to safety evaluations should be reported to the sponsor according to the reporting requirements and within the time periods specified by the sponsor in the protocol.

4.11.3 For reported deaths, the investigator should supply the sponsor and the IRB/IEC with any additional requested information (e.g., autopsy reports and terminal medical reports).

4.12 *Premature Termination or Suspension of a Trial*

If the trial is terminated prematurely or suspended for any reason, the investigator/institution should promptly inform the trial subjects, should assure appropriate therapy and follow-up for the subjects, and, where required by the applicable regulatory requirement(s), should inform the regulatory authority(ies). In addition:

4.12.1 If the investigator terminates or suspends a trial without prior agreement of the sponsor, the investigator should inform the institution, where required by the applicable regulatory requirements, and the investigator/institution should promptly inform the sponsor and the IRB/IEC, and should provide the sponsor and the IRB/IEC a detailed written explanation of the termination or suspension.

4.12.2 If the sponsor terminates or suspends a trial (see 5.21), the investigator should

promptly inform the institution, where required by the applicable regulatory requirements, and the investigator/institution should promptly inform the IRB/IEC and provide the IRB/IEC a detailed written explanation of the termination or suspension.

4.12.3 If the IRB/IEC terminates or suspends its approval/favorable opinion of a trial (see 3.1.2 and 3.3.9), the investigator should inform the institution, where required by the applicable regulatory requirements, and the investigator/institution should promptly notify the sponsor and provide the sponsor with a detailed written explanation of the termination or suspension.

4.13 *Final Report(s) by Investigator/ Institution*

Upon completion of the trial, the investigator should, where required by the applicable regulatory requirements, inform the institution, and the investigator/ institution should provide the sponsor with all required reports, the IRB/IEC with a summary of the trial's outcome, and the regulatory authority(ies) with any report(s) they require of the investigator/institution.

5. *Sponsor*

5.1 *Quality Assurance and Quality Control*

5.1.1 The sponsor is responsible for implementing and maintaining quality assurance and quality control systems with written SOP's to ensure that trials are conducted and data are generated, documented (recorded), and reported in compliance with the protocol, GCP, and the applicable regulatory requirement(s).

5.1.2 The sponsor is responsible for securing agreement from all involved parties to ensure direct access (see 1.21) to all trial-related sites, source data/documents, and reports for the purpose of monitoring and auditing by the sponsor, and inspection by domestic and foreign regulatory authorities.

5.1.3 Quality control should be applied to each stage of data handling to ensure that all data are reliable and have been processed correctly.

5.1.4 Agreements, made by the sponsor with the investigator/institution and/or with any other parties involved with the clinical trial, should be in writing, as part of the protocol or in a separate agreement.

5.2 *Contract Research Organization (CRO)*

5.2.1 A sponsor may transfer any or all of the sponsor's trial-related duties and functions to a CRO, but the ultimate responsibility for the quality and integrity of the trial data always resides with the sponsor. The CRO should implement quality assurance and quality control.

5.2.2 Any trial-related duty and function that is transferred to and assumed by a CRO should be specified in writing.

5.2.3 Any trial-related duties and functions not specifically transferred to and assumed by a CRO are retained by the sponsor.

5.2.4 All references to a sponsor in this guideline also apply to a CRO to the extent that a CRO has assumed the trial-related duties and functions of a sponsor.

5.3 *Medical Expertise*

The sponsor should designate appropriately qualified medical personnel who will be readily available to advise on trial-related medical questions or problems. If necessary, outside consultant(s) may be appointed for this purpose.

5.4 *Trial Design*

5.4.1 The sponsor should utilize qualified individuals (e.g., biostatisticians, clinical pharmacologists, and physicians) as appropriate, throughout all stages of the trial process, from designing the protocol and CRF's and planning the analyses to analyzing and preparing interim and final clinical trial/ study reports.

5.4.2 For further guidance: Clinical Trial Protocol and Protocol Amendment(s) (see 6.), the ICH Guideline for Structure and Content of Clinical Study Reports, and other appropriate ICH guidance on trial design, protocol, and conduct.

5.5 *Trial Management, Data Handling, Recordkeeping, and Independent Data Monitoring Committee*

5.5.1 The sponsor should utilize appropriately qualified individuals to supervise the overall conduct of the trial, to handle the data, to verify the data, to conduct the statistical analyses, and to prepare the trial reports.

5.5.2 The sponsor may consider establishing an independent data monitoring committee (IDMC) to assess the progress of a clinical trial, including the safety data and the critical efficacy endpoints at intervals, and to recommend to the sponsor whether to continue, modify, or stop a trial. The IDMC should have written operating procedures and maintain written records of all its meetings.

5.5.3 When using electronic trial data handling and/or remote electronic trial data systems, the sponsor should:

(a) Ensure and document that the electronic data processing system(s) conforms to the sponsor's established requirements for completeness, accuracy, reliability, and consistent intended performance (i.e., validation).

(b) Maintain SOP's for using these systems.

(c) Ensure that the systems are designed to permit data changes in such a way that the data changes are documented and that there is no deletion of entered data (i.e., maintain an audit trail, data trail, edit trail).

(d) Maintain a security system that prevents unauthorized access to the data.

(e) Maintain a list of the individuals who are authorized to make data changes (see 4.1.5 and 4.9.3).

(f) Maintain adequate backup of the data.

(g) Safeguard the blinding, if any (e.g., maintain the blinding during data entry and processing).

5.5.4 If data are transformed during processing, it should always be possible to compare the original data and observations with the processed data.

5.5.5 The sponsor should use an unambiguous subject identification code (see 1.58) that allows identification of all the data reported for each subject.

5.5.6 The sponsor, or other owners of the data, should retain all of the sponsor-specific essential documents pertaining to the trial. (See 8. "Essential Documents for the Conduct of a Clinical Trial.")

5.5.7 The sponsor should retain all sponsor-specific essential documents in conformance with the applicable regulatory requirement(s) of the country(ies) where the product is approved, and/or where the sponsor intends to apply for approval(s).

5.5.8 If the sponsor discontinues the clinical development of an investigational product (i.e., for any or all indications, routes of administration, or dosage forms), the sponsor should maintain all sponsor-specific essential documents for at least 2 years after formal discontinuation or in conformance with the applicable regulatory requirement(s).

5.5.9 If the sponsor discontinues the clinical development of an investigational product, the sponsor should notify all the trial investigators/institutions and all the appropriate regulatory authorities.

5.5.10 Any transfer of ownership of the data should be reported to the appropriate authority(ies), as required by the applicable regulatory requirement(s).

5.5.11 The sponsor-specific essential documents should be retained until at least 2 years after the last approval of a marketing application in an ICH region and until there are no pending or contemplated marketing applications in an ICH region or at least 2 years have elapsed since the formal discontinuation of clinical development of the investigational product. These documents should be retained for a longer period, however, if required by the applicable regulatory requirement(s) or if needed by the sponsor.

5.5.12 The sponsor should inform the investigator(s)/institution(s) in writing of the need for record retention and should notify the investigator(s)/institution(s) in writing when the trial-related records are no longer needed (see 4.9.5).

5.6 *Investigator Selection*

5.6.1 The sponsor is responsible for selecting the investigator(s)/institution(s). Each investigator should be qualified by training and experience and should have adequate resources (see 4.1, 4.2) to properly conduct the trial for which the investigator is selected. If a coordinating committee and/or coordinating investigator(s) are to be utilized in multicenter trials, their organization and/ or selection are the sponsor's responsibility.

5.6.2 Before entering an agreement with an investigator/institution to conduct a trial, the sponsor should provide the investigator(s)/ institution(s) with the protocol and an up-to-date Investigator's Brochure, and should provide sufficient time for the investigator/ institution to review the protocol and the information provided.

5.6.3 The sponsor should obtain the investigator's/institution's agreement:

(a) To conduct the trial in compliance with GCP, with the applicable regulatory requirement(s), and with the protocol agreed to by the sponsor and given approval/ favorable opinion by the IRB/IEC;

(b) To comply with procedures for data recording/reporting; and

(c) To permit monitoring, auditing, and inspection (see 4.1.4).

(d) To retain the essential documents that should be in the investigator/institution files (see 8.) until the sponsor informs the investigator/institution these documents are no longer needed (see 4.9.4, 4.9.5, and 5.5.12).

The sponsor and the investigator/ institution should sign the protocol, or an alternative document, to confirm this agreement.

5.7 *Allocation of Duties and Functions*

Prior to initiating a trial, the sponsor should define, establish, and allocate all trial-related duties and functions.

5.8 *Compensation to Subjects and Investigators*

5.8.1 If required by the applicable regulatory requirement(s), the sponsor should provide insurance or should indemnify (legal and financial coverage) the investigator/the institution against claims arising from the trial, except for claims that arise from malpractice and/or negligence.

5.8.2 The sponsor's policies and procedures should address the costs of treatment of trial subjects in the event of trial-related injuries in accordance with the applicable regulatory requirement(s).

5.8.3 When trial subjects receive compensation, the method and manner of compensation should comply with applicable regulatory requirement(s).

5.9 *Financing*

The financial aspects of the trial should be documented in an agreement between the sponsor and the investigator/institution.

5.10 *Notification/Submission to Regulatory Authority(ies)*

Before initiating the clinical trial(s), the sponsor (or the sponsor and the investigator, if required by the applicable regulatory requirement(s)), should submit any required application(s) to the appropriate authority(ies) for review, acceptance, and/or permission (as required by the applicable regulatory requirement(s)) to begin the trial(s). Any notification/submission should be dated and contain sufficient information to identify the protocol.

5.11 *Confirmation of Review by IRB/IEC*

5.11.1 The sponsor should obtain from the investigator/institution:

(a) The name and address of the investigator's/institution's IRB/IEC.

(b) A statement obtained from the IRB/IEC that it is organized and operates according to GCP and the applicable laws and regulations.

(c) Documented IRB/IEC approval/ favorable opinion and, if requested by the sponsor, a current copy of protocol, written informed consent form(s) and any other written information to be provided to subjects, subject recruiting procedures, and documents related to payments and compensation available to the subjects, and any other documents that the IRB/IEC may have requested.

5.11.2 If the IRB/IEC conditions its approval/ favorable opinion upon change(s) in any aspect of the trial, such as modification(s) of the protocol, written informed consent form and any other written information to be provided to subjects, and/or other procedures, the sponsor should obtain from the investigator/institution a copy of the modification(s) made and the date approval/ favorable opinion was given by the IRB/IEC.

5.11.3 The sponsor should obtain from the investigator/institution documentation and dates of any IRB/IEC reapprovals/ reevaluations with favorable opinion, and of any withdrawals or suspensions of approval/ favorable opinion.

5.12 *Information on Investigational Product(s)*

5.12.1 When planning trials, the sponsor should ensure that sufficient safety and efficacy data from nonclinical studies and/or clinical trials are available to support human exposure by the route, at the dosages, for the duration, and in the trial population to be studied.

5.12.2 The sponsor should update the Investigator's Brochure as significant new information becomes available. (See 7. "Investigator's Brochure.")

5.13 *Manufacturing, Packaging, Labeling, and Coding Investigational Product(s)*

5.13.1 The sponsor should ensure that the investigational product(s) (including active comparator(s) and placebo, if applicable) is characterized as appropriate to the stage of development of the product(s), is manufactured in accordance with any applicable GMP, and is coded and labeled in a manner that protects the blinding, if applicable. In addition, the labeling should comply with applicable regulatory requirement(s).

5.13.2 The sponsor should determine, for the investigational product(s), acceptable storage temperatures, storage conditions (e.g., protection from light), storage times, reconstitution fluids and procedures, and devices for product infusion, if any. The sponsor should inform all involved parties (e.g., monitors, investigators, pharmacists, storage managers) of these determinations.

5.13.3 The investigational product(s) should be packaged to prevent contamination and unacceptable deterioration during transport and storage.

5.13.4 In blinded trials, the coding system for the investigational product(s) should include a mechanism that permits rapid identification of the product(s) in case of a medical emergency, but does not permit undetectable breaks of the blinding.

5.13.5 If significant formulation changes are made in the investigational or comparator product(s) during the course of clinical development, the results of any additional studies of the formulated product(s) (e.g., stability, dissolution rate, bioavailability) needed to assess whether these changes would significantly alter the pharmacokinetic profile of the product should be available prior to the use of the new formulation in clinical trials.

5.14 *Supplying and Handling Investigational Product(s)*

5.14.1 The sponsor is responsible for supplying the investigator(s)/institution(s) with the investigational product(s).

5.14.2 The sponsor should not supply an investigator/institution with the investigational product(s) until the sponsor obtains all required documentation (e.g., approval/favorable opinion from IRB/IEC and regulatory authority(ies)).

5.14.3 The sponsor should ensure that written procedures include instructions that the investigator/institution should follow for the handling and storage of investigational product(s) for the trial and documentation thereof. The procedures should address adequate and safe receipt, handling, storage, dispensing, retrieval of unused product from subjects, and return of unused investigational product(s) to the sponsor (or alternative disposition if authorized by the sponsor and in compliance with the applicable regulatory requirement(s)).

5.14.4 The sponsor should:

(a) Ensure timely delivery of investigational product(s) to the investigator(s).

(b) Maintain records that document shipment, receipt, disposition, return, and destruction of the investigational product(s). (See 8. "Essential Documents for the Conduct of a Clinical Trial.")

(c) Maintain a system for retrieving investigational products and documenting this retrieval (e.g., for deficient product recall, reclaim after trial completion, expired product reclaim).

(d) Maintain a system for the disposition of unused investigational product(s) and for the documentation of this disposition.

5.14.5 The sponsor should:

(a) Take steps to ensure that the investigational product(s) are stable over the period of use.

(b) Maintain sufficient quantities of the investigational product(s) used in the trials to reconfirm specifications, should this become necessary, and maintain records of batch sample analyses and characteristics. To the extent stability permits, samples should be retained either until the analyses of the trial data are complete or as required by the applicable regulatory requirement(s), whichever represents the longer retention period.

5.15 *Record Access*

5.15.1 The sponsor should ensure that it is specified in the protocol or other written agreement that the investigator(s)/ institution(s) provide direct access to source data/documents for trial-related monitoring, audits, IRB/IEC review, and regulatory inspection.

5.15.2 The sponsor should verify that each subject has consented, in writing, to direct access to his/her original medical records for trial-related monitoring, audit, IRB/IEC review, and regulatory inspection.

5.16 *Safety Information*

5.16.1 The sponsor is responsible for the ongoing safety evaluation of the investigational product(s).

5.16.2 The sponsor should promptly notify all concerned investigator(s)/institution(s) and the regulatory authority(ies) of findings that could affect adversely the safety of subjects, impact the conduct of the trial, or alter the IRB/IEC's approval/favorable opinion to continue the trial.

5.17 *Adverse Drug Reaction Reporting*

5.17.1 The sponsor should expedite the reporting to all concerned investigator(s)/ institutions(s), to the IRB(s)/IEC(s), where required, and to the regulatory authority(ies) of all adverse drug reactions (ADR's) that are both serious and unexpected.

5.17.2 Such expedited reports should comply with the applicable regulatory requirement(s) and with the ICH Guideline for Clinical Safety Data Management: Definitions and Standards for Expedited Reporting.

5.17.3 The sponsor should submit to the regulatory authority(ies) all safety updates and periodic reports, as required by applicable regulatory requirement(s).

5.18 *Monitoring*

5.18.1 *Purpose*. The purposes of trial monitoring are to verify that:

(a) The rights and well-being of human subjects are protected.

(b) The reported trial data are accurate, complete, and verifiable from source documents.

(c) The conduct of the trial is in compliance with the currently approved protocol/amendment(s), with GCP, and with applicable regulatory requirement(s).

5.18.2 *Selection and Qualifications of Monitors.*

(a) Monitors should be appointed by the sponsor.

(b) Monitors should be appropriately trained, and should have the scientific and/ or clinical knowledge needed to monitor the trial adequately. A monitor's qualifications should be documented.

(c) Monitors should be thoroughly familiar with the investigational product(s), the protocol, written informed consent form and any other written information to be provided to subjects, the sponsor's SOP's, GCP, and the applicable regulatory requirement(s).

5.18.3 *Extent and Nature of Monitoring.*

The sponsor should ensure that the trials are adequately monitored. The sponsor should determine the appropriate extent and nature of monitoring. The determination of the extent and nature of monitoring should be based on considerations such as the objective, purpose, design, complexity, blinding, size, and endpoints of the trial. In general there is a need for on-site monitoring, before, during, and after the trial; however, in exceptional circumstances the sponsor may determine that central monitoring in conjunction with procedures such as investigators' training and meetings, and extensive written guidance can assure appropriate conduct of the trial in accordance with GCP. Statistically controlled sampling may be an acceptable method for selecting the data to be verified.

5.18.4 *Monitor's Responsibilities.*

The monitor(s), in accordance with the sponsor's requirements, should ensure that the trial is conducted and documented properly by carrying out the following activities when relevant and necessary to the trial and the trial site:

(a) Acting as the main line of communication between the sponsor and the investigator.

(b) Verifying that the investigator has adequate qualifications and resources (see 4.1, 4.2, 5.6) and these remain adequate throughout the trial period, and that the staff and facilities, including laboratories and equipment, are adequate to safely and properly conduct the trial and these remain adequate throughout the trial period.

(c) Verifying, for the investigational product(s):

(i) That storage times and conditions are acceptable, and that supplies are sufficient throughout the trial.

(ii) That the investigational product(s) are supplied only to subjects who are eligible to receive it and at the protocol specified dose(s).

(iii) That subjects are provided with necessary instruction on properly using, handling, storing, and returning the investigational product(s).

(iv) That the receipt, use, and return of the investigational product(s) at the trial sites are controlled and documented adequately.

(v) That the disposition of unused investigational product(s) at the trial sites complies with applicable regulatory requirement(s) and is in accordance with the sponsor's authorized procedures.

(d) Verifying that the investigator follows the approved protocol and all approved amendment(s), if any.

(e) Verifying that written informed consent was obtained before each subject's participation in the trial.

(f) Ensuring that the investigator receives the current Investigator's Brochure, all documents, and all trial supplies needed to conduct the trial properly and to comply with the applicable regulatory requirement(s).

(g) Ensuring that the investigator and the investigator's trial staff are adequately informed about the trial.

(h) Verifying that the investigator and the investigator's trial staff are performing the specified trial functions, in accordance with the protocol and any other written agreement between the sponsor and the investigator/ institution, and have not delegated these functions to unauthorized individuals.

(i) Verifying that the investigator is enrolling only eligible subjects.

(j) Reporting the subject recruitment rate.

(k) Verifying that source data/documents and other trial records are accurate, complete, kept up-to-date, and maintained.

(l) Verifying that the investigator provides all the required reports, notifications, applications, and submissions, and that these documents are accurate, complete, timely, legible, dated, and identify the trial.

(m) Checking the accuracy and completeness of the CRF entries, source data/ documents, and other trial-related records against each other. The monitor specifically should verify that:

(i) The data required by the protocol are reported accurately on the CRF's and are consistent with the source data/documents.

(ii) Any dose and/or therapy modifications are well documented for each of the trial subjects.

(iii) Adverse events, concomitant medications, and intercurrent illnesses are reported in accordance with the protocol on the CRF's.

(iv) Visits that the subjects fail to make, tests that are not conducted, and examinations that are not performed are clearly reported as such on the CRF's.

(v) All withdrawals and dropouts of enrolled subjects from the trial are reported and explained on the CRF's.

(n) Informing the investigator of any CRF entry error, omission, or illegibility. The monitor should ensure that appropriate corrections, additions, or deletions are made, dated, explained (if necessary), and initialed by the investigator or by a member of the investigator's trial staff who is authorized to initial CRF changes for the investigator. This authorization should be documented.

(o) Determining whether all adverse events (AE's) are appropriately reported within the time periods required by GCP, the protocol, the IRB/IEC, the sponsor, the applicable regulatory requirement(s), and indicated in the ICH Guideline for Clinical Safety Data Management: Definitions and Standards for Expedited Reporting.

(p) Determining whether the investigator is maintaining the essential documents. (See 8. "Essential Documents for the Conduct of a Clinical Trial.")

(q) Communicating deviations from the protocol, SOP's, GCP, and the applicable regulatory requirements to the investigator and taking appropriate action designed to prevent recurrence of the detected deviations.

5.18.5 *Monitoring Procedures.*

The monitor(s) should follow the sponsor's established written SOP's as well as those procedures that are specified by the sponsor for monitoring a specific trial.

5.18.6 *Monitoring Report.*

(a) The monitor should submit a written report to the sponsor after each trial-site visit or trial-related communication.

(b) Reports should include the date, site, name of the monitor, and name of the investigator or other individual(s) contacted.

(c) Reports should include a summary of what the monitor reviewed and the monitor's statements concerning the significant findings/facts, deviations and deficiencies, conclusions, actions taken or to be taken, and/or actions recommended to secure compliance.

(d) The review and follow-up of the monitoring report by the sponsor should be documented by the sponsor's designated representative.

5.19 *Audit*

If or when sponsors perform audits, as part of implementing quality assurance, they should consider:

5.19.1 *Purpose.*

The purpose of a sponsor's audit, which is independent of and separate from routine monitoring or quality control functions, should be to evaluate trial conduct and compliance with the protocol, SOP's, GCP, and the applicable regulatory requirements.

5.19.2 *Selection and Qualification of Auditors.*

(a) The sponsor should appoint individuals, who are independent of the clinical trial/data collection system(s), to conduct audits.

(b) The sponsor should ensure that the auditors are qualified by training and experience to conduct audits properly. An auditor's qualifications should be documented.

5.19.3 *Auditing Procedures.*

(a) The sponsor should ensure that the auditing of clinical trials/systems is conducted in accordance with the sponsor's written procedures on what to audit, how to audit, the frequency of audits, and the form and content of audit reports.

(b) The sponsor's audit plan and procedures for a trial audit should be guided by the importance of the trial to submissions to regulatory authorities, the number of subjects in the trial, the type and complexity of the trial, the level of risks to the trial subjects, and any identified problem(s).

(c) The observations and findings of the auditor(s) should be documented.

(d) To preserve the independence and value of the audit function, the regulatory authority(ies) should not routinely request the audit reports. Regulatory authority(ies) may seek access to an audit report on a case-by-case basis, when evidence of serious GCP noncompliance exists, or in the course of legal proceedings or investigations.

(e) Where required by applicable law or regulation, the sponsor should provide an audit certificate.

5.20 *Noncompliance*

5.20.1 Noncompliance with the protocol, SOP's, GCP, and/or applicable regulatory requirement(s) by an investigator/institution, or by member(s) of the sponsor's staff should lead to prompt action by the sponsor to secure compliance.

5.20.2 If the monitoring and/or auditing identifies serious and/or persistent noncompliance on the part of an investigator/institution, the sponsor should terminate the investigator's/institution's participation in the trial. When an investigator's/institution's participation is terminated because of noncompliance, the sponsor should notify promptly the regulatory authority(ies).

5.21 *Premature Termination or Suspension of a Trial*

If a trial is terminated prematurely or suspended, the sponsor should promptly inform the investigators/institutions, and the regulatory authority(ies) of the termination or suspension and the reason(s) for the termination or suspension. The IRB/IEC should also be informed promptly and provided the reason(s) for the termination or suspension by the sponsor or by the investigator/institution, as specified by the applicable regulatory requirement(s).

5.22 *Clinical Trial/Study Reports*

Whether the trial is completed or prematurely terminated, the sponsor should ensure that the clinical trial/study reports are prepared and provided to the regulatory agency(ies) as required by the applicable regulatory requirement(s). The sponsor should also ensure that the clinical trial/study reports in marketing applications meet the standards of the ICH Guideline for Structure and Content of Clinical Study Reports. (NOTE: The ICH Guideline for Structure and Content of Clinical Study Reports specifies that abbreviated study reports may be acceptable in certain cases.)

5.23 *Multicenter Trials*

For multicenter trials, the sponsor should ensure that:

5.23.1 All investigators conduct the trial in strict compliance with the protocol agreed to by the sponsor and, if required, by the regulatory authority(ies), and given approval/favorable opinion by the IRB/IEC.

5.23.2 The CRF's are designed to capture the required data at all multicenter trial sites. For those investigators who are collecting additional data, supplemental CRF's should also be provided that are designed to capture the additional data.

5.23.3 The responsibilities of the coordinating investigator(s) and the other participating investigators are documented prior to the start of the trial.

5.23.4 All investigators are given instructions on following the protocol, on complying with a uniform set of standards for the assessment of clinical and laboratory findings, and on completing the CRF's.

5.23.5 Communication between investigators is facilitated.

6. *Clinical Trial Protocol and Protocol Amendment(s)*

The contents of a trial protocol should generally include the following topics. However, site specific information may be provided on separate protocol page(s), or addressed in a separate agreement, and some of the information listed below may be contained in other protocol referenced documents, such as an Investigator's Brochure.

6.1 *General Information*

6.1.1 Protocol title, protocol identifying number, and date. Any amendment(s) should also bear the amendment number(s) and date(s).

6.1.2 Name and address of the sponsor and monitor (if other than the sponsor).

6.1.3 Name and title of the person(s) authorized to sign the protocol and the protocol amendment(s) for the sponsor.

6.1.4 Name, title, address, and telephone number(s) of the sponsor's medical expert (or dentist when appropriate) for the trial.

6.1.5 Name and title of the investigator(s) who is (are) responsible for conducting the trial, and the address and telephone number(s) of the trial site(s).

6.1.6 Name, title, address, and telephone number(s) of the qualified physician (or dentist, if applicable) who is responsible for all trial-site related medical (or dental) decisions (if other than investigator).

6.1.7 Name(s) and address(es) of the clinical laboratory(ies) and other medical and/or technical department(s) and/or institutions involved in the trial.

6.2 *Background Information*

6.2.1 Name and description of the investigational product(s).

6.2.2 A summary of findings from nonclinical studies that potentially have clinical significance and from clinical trials that are relevant to the trial.

6.2.3 Summary of the known and potential risks and benefits, if any, to human subjects.

6.2.4 Description of and justification for the route of administration, dosage, dosage regimen, and treatment period(s).

6.2.5 A statement that the trial will be conducted in compliance with the protocol, GCP, and the applicable regulatory requirement(s).

6.2.6 Description of the population to be studied.

6.2.7 References to literature and data that are relevant to the trial, and that provide background for the trial.

6.3 *Trial Objectives and Purpose*

A detailed description of the objectives and the purpose of the trial.

6.4 *Trial Design*

The scientific integrity of the trial and the credibility of the data from the trial depend substantially on the trial design. A description of the trial design should include:

6.4.1 A specific statement of the primary endpoints and the secondary endpoints, if any, to be measured during the trial.

6.4.2 A description of the type/design of trial to be conducted (e.g., double-blind, placebo-controlled, parallel design) and a schematic diagram of trial design, procedures, and stages.

6.4.3 A description of the measures taken to minimize/avoid bias, including (for example):

(a) Randomization.

(b) Blinding.

6.4.4 A description of the trial treatment(s) and the dosage and dosage regimen of the investigational product(s). Also include a description of the dosage form, packaging, and labeling of the investigational product(s).

6.4.5 The expected duration of subject participation, and a description of the sequence and duration of all trial periods, including follow-up, if any.

6.4.6 A description of the "stopping rules" or "discontinuation criteria" for individual subjects, parts of trial, and entire trial.

6.4.7 Accountability procedures for the investigational product(s), including the placebo(s) and comparator(s), if any.

6.4.8 Maintenance of trial treatment randomization codes and procedures for breaking codes.

6.4.9 The identification of any data to be recorded directly on the CRF's (i.e., no prior written or electronic record of data), and to be considered to be source data.

6.5 *Selection and Withdrawal of Subjects*

6.5.1 Subject inclusion criteria.

6.5.2 Subject exclusion criteria.

6.5.3 Subject withdrawal criteria (i.e., terminating investigational product treatment/trial treatment) and procedures specifying:

(a) When and how to withdraw subjects from the trial/ investigational product treatment.

(b) The type and timing of the data to be collected for withdrawn subjects.

(c) Whether and how subjects are to be replaced.

(d) The follow-up for subjects withdrawn from investigational product treatment/trial treatment.

6.6 *Treatment of Subjects*

6.6.1 The treatment(s) to be administered, including the name(s) of all the product(s), the dose(s), the dosing schedule(s), the route/ mode(s) of administration, and the treatment period(s), including the follow-up period(s) for subjects for each investigational product treatment/trial treatment group/arm of the trial.

6.6.2 Medication(s)/treatment(s) permitted (including rescue medication) and not permitted before and/or during the trial.

6.6.3 Procedures for monitoring subject compliance.

6.7 *Assessment of Efficacy*

6.7.1 Specification of the efficacy parameters.

6.7.2 Methods and timing for assessing, recording, and analyzing efficacy parameters.

6.8 *Assessment of Safety*

6.8.1 Specification of safety parameters.

6.8.2 The methods and timing for assessing, recording, and analyzing safety parameters.

6.8.3 Procedures for eliciting reports of and for recording and reporting adverse event and intercurrent illnesses.

6.8.4 The type and duration of the follow-up of subjects after adverse events.

6.9 *Statistics*

6.9.1 A description of the statistical methods to be employed, including timing of any planned interim analysis(ses).

6.9.2 The number of subjects planned to be enrolled. In multicenter trials, the number of enrolled subjects projected for each trial site should be specified. Reason for choice of sample size, including reflections on (or calculations of) the power of the trial and clinical justification.

6.9.3 The level of significance to be used.

6.9.4 Criteria for the termination of the trial.

6.9.5 Procedure for accounting for missing, unused, and spurious data.

6.9.6 Procedures for reporting any deviation(s) from the original statistical plan (any deviation(s) from the original statistical plan should be described and justified in the protocol and/or in the final report, as appropriate).

6.9.7 The selection of subjects to be included in the analyses (e.g., all randomized subjects, all dosed subjects, all eligible subjects, evaluate-able subjects).

6.10 *Direct Access to Source Data/Documents*

The sponsor should ensure that it is specified in the protocol or other written agreement that the investigator(s)/ institution(s) will permit trial-related monitoring, audits, IRB/IEC review, and regulatory inspection(s) by providing direct access to source data/documents.

6.11 *Quality Control and Quality Assurance*

6.12 *Ethics*

Description of ethical considerations relating to the trial.

6.13 *Data Handling and Recordkeeping*

6.14 *Financing and Insurance*

Financing and insurance if not addressed in a separate agreement.

6.15 *Publication Policy*

Publication policy, if not addressed in a separate agreement.

6.16 *Supplements*

(NOTE: Since the protocol and the clinical trial/study report are closely related, further relevant information can be found in the ICH Guideline for Structure and Content of Clinical Study Reports.)

7. *Investigator's Brochure*

7.1 *Introduction*

The Investigator's Brochure (IB) is a compilation of the clinical and nonclinical data on the investigational product(s) that are relevant to the study of the product(s) in human subjects. Its purpose is to provide the investigators and others involved in the trial with the information to facilitate their understanding of the rationale for, and their compliance with, many key features of the protocol, such as the dose, dose frequency/ interval, methods of administration, and safety monitoring procedures. The IB also provides insight to support the clinical management of the study subjects during the course of the clinical trial. The information should be presented in a concise, simple, objective, balanced, and nonpromotional form that enables a clinician, or potential investigator, to understand it and make his/ her own unbiased risk-benefit assessment of the appropriateness of the proposed trial. For this reason, a medically qualified person should generally participate in the editing of an IB, but the contents of the IB should be approved by the disciplines that generated the described data.

This guideline delineates the minimum information that should be included in an IB and provides suggestions for its layout. It is expected that the type and extent of information available will vary with the stage of development of the investigational product. If the investigational product is marketed and its pharmacology is widely understood by medical practitioners, an extensive IB may not be necessary. Where permitted by regulatory authorities, a basic product information brochure, package leaflet, or labeling may be an appropriate alternative, provided that it includes current, comprehensive, and detailed information on all aspects of the investigational product that might be of importance to the investigator. If a marketed product is being studied for a new use (i.e., a new indication), an IB specific to that new use should be prepared. The IB should be reviewed at least annually and revised as necessary in compliance with a sponsor's written procedures. More frequent revision may be appropriate depending on the stage of development and the generation of relevant new information. However, in accordance with GCP, relevant new information may be so important that it should be communicated to the investigators, and possibly to the Institutional Review Boards (IRB's)/Independent Ethics Committees (IEC's) and/or regulatory authorities before it is included in a revised IB.

Generally, the sponsor is responsible for ensuring that an up-to-date IB is made available to the investigator(s) and the investigators are responsible for providing the up-to-date IB to the responsible IRB's/ IEC's. In the case of an investigator-sponsored trial, the sponsor-investigator should determine whether a brochure is available from the commercial manufacturer. If the investigational product is provided by the sponsor-investigator, then he or she should provide the necessary information to the trial personnel. In cases where preparation of a formal IB is impractical, the sponsor-investigator should provide, as a substitute, an expanded background information section in the trial protocol that contains the minimum current information described in this guideline.

7.2 *General Considerations*

The IB should include:

7.2.1 *Title Page.* This should provide the sponsor's name, the identity of each investigational product (i.e., research number, chemical or approved generic name, and trade name(s) where legally permissible and desired by the sponsor), and the release date. It is also suggested that an edition number, and a reference to the number and date of the edition it supersedes, be provided. An example is given in Appendix 1.

7.2.2 *Confidentiality Statement.* The sponsor may wish to include a statement instructing the investigator/recipients to treat the IB as a confidential document for the sole information and use of the investigator's team and the IRB/IEC.

7.3 *Contents of the Investigator's Brochure.* The IB should contain the following sections, each with literature references where appropriate:

7.3.1 *Table of Contents.* An example of the Table of Contents is given in Appendix 2.

7.3.2 *Summary.* A brief summary (preferably not exceeding two pages) should be given, highlighting the significant physical, chemical, pharmaceutical, pharmacological, toxicological, pharmacokinetic, metabolic, and clinical information available that is relevant to the stage of clinical development of the investigational product.

7.3.3 *Introduction.*   A brief introductory statement should be provided that contains the chemical name (and generic and trade name(s) when approved) of the investigational product(s), all active ingredients, the investigational product(s) pharmacological class and its expected position within this class (e.g., advantages), the rationale for performing research with the investigational product(s), and the anticipated prophylactic, therapeutic, or diagnostic indication(s). Finally, the introductory statement should provide the general approach to be followed in evaluating the investigational product.

7.3.4 *Physical, Chemical, and Pharmaceutical Properties and Formulation.* A description should be provided of the investigational product substance(s) (including the chemical and/or structural formula(e)), and a brief summary should be given of the relevant physical, chemical, and pharmaceutical properties.

To permit appropriate safety measures to be taken in the course of the trial, a description of the formulation(s) to be used, including excipients, should be provided and justified if clinically relevant. Instructions for the storage and handling of the dosage form(s) should also be given.

Any structural similarities to other known compounds should be mentioned.

7.3.5 *Nonclinical Studies.*

Introduction:

The results of all relevant nonclinical pharmacology, toxicology, pharmacokinetic, and investigational product metabolism studies should be provided in summary form. This summary should address the methodology used, the results, and a discussion of the relevance of the findings to the investigated therapeutic and the possible unfavorable and unintended effects in humans.

The information provided may include the following, as appropriate, if known/available:

Species tested;

Number and sex of animals in each group;

Unit dose (e.g., milligram/kilogram (mg/ kg));

Dose interval;

Route of administration;

Duration of dosing;

Information on systemic distribution;

Duration of post-exposure follow-up;

Results, including the following aspects:

- Nature and frequency of pharmacological or toxic effects;

- Severity or intensity of pharmacological or toxic effects;

- Time to onset of effects;

- Reversibility of effects;

- Duration of effects;

- Dose response.

Tabular format/listings should be used whenever possible to enhance the clarity of the presentation.

The following sections should discuss the most important findings from the studies, including the dose response of observed effects, the relevance to humans, and any aspects to be studied in humans. If applicable, the effective and nontoxic dose

findings in the same animal species should be compared (i.e., the therapeutic index should be discussed). The relevance of this information to the proposed human dosing should be addressed. Whenever possible, comparisons should be made in terms of blood/tissue levels rather than on a mg/kg basis.

(a) Nonclinical Pharmacology

A summary of the pharmacological aspects of the investigational product and, where appropriate, its significant metabolites studied in animals should be included. Such a summary should incorporate studies that assess potential therapeutic activity (e.g., efficacy models, receptor binding, and specificity) as well as those that assess safety (e.g., special studies to assess pharmacological actions other than the intended therapeutic effect(s)).

(b) Pharmacokinetics and Product Metabolism in Animals

A summary of the pharmacokinetics and biological transformation and disposition of the investigational product in all species studied should be given. The discussion of the findings should address the absorption and the local and systemic bioavailability of the investigational product and its metabolites, and their relationship to the pharmacological and toxicological findings in animal species.

(c) Toxicology

A summary of the toxicological effects found in relevant studies conducted in different animal species should be described under the following headings where appropriate:

Single dose;

Repeated dose;

Carcinogenicity;

Special studies (e.g., irritancy and sensitization);

Reproductive toxicity;

Genotoxicity (mutagenicity).

7.3.6 *Effects in Humans.*

Introduction:

A thorough discussion of the known effects of the investigational product(s) in humans should be provided, including information on pharmacokinetics, metabolism, pharmacodynamics, dose response, safety, efficacy, and other pharmacological activities. Where possible, a summary of each completed clinical trial should be provided. Information should also be provided regarding results from any use of the investigational product(s) other than in clinical trials, such as from experience during marketing.

(a) Pharmacokinetics and Product Metabolism in Humans

A summary of information on the pharmacokinetics of the investigational product(s) should be presented, including the following, if available:

Pharmacokinetics (including metabolism, as appropriate, and absorption, plasma protein binding, distribution, and elimination).

Bioavailability of the investigational product (absolute, where possible, and/or relative) using a reference dosage form.

Population subgroups (e.g., gender, age, and impaired organ function).

Interactions (e.g., product-product interactions and effects of food).

Other pharmacokinetic data (e.g., results of population studies performed within clinical trial(s)).

(b) Safety and Efficacy

A summary of information should be provided about the investigational product's/ products' (including metabolites, where appropriate) safety, pharmacodynamics, efficacy, and dose response that were obtained from preceding trials in humans (healthy volunteers and/or patients). The implications of this information should be discussed. In cases where a number of clinical trials have been completed, the use of summaries of safety and efficacy across multiple trials by indications in subgroups may provide a clear presentation of the data. Tabular summaries of adverse drug reactions for all the clinical trials (including those for all the studied indications) would be useful. Important differences in adverse drug reaction patterns/incidences across indications or subgroups should be discussed.

The IB should provide a description of the possible risks and adverse drug reactions to be anticipated on the basis of prior experiences with the product under investigation and with related products. A description should also be provided of the precautions or special monitoring to be done as part of the investigational use of the product(s).

(c) Marketing Experience

The IB should identify countries where the investigational product has been marketed or approved. Any significant information arising from the marketed use should be summarized (e.g., formulations, dosages, routes of administration, and adverse product reactions). The IB should also identify all the countries where the investigational product did not receive approval/registration for marketing or was withdrawn from marketing/ registration.

7.3.7 *Summary of Data and Guidance for the Investigator.*

This section should provide an overall discussion of the nonclinical and clinical data, and should summarize the information from various sources on different aspects of the investigational product(s), wherever possible. In this way, the investigator can be provided with the most informative interpretation of the available data and with an assessment of the implications of the information for future clinical trials.

Where appropriate, the published reports on related products should be discussed. This could help the investigator to anticipate adverse drug reactions or other problems in clinical trials.

The overall aim of this section is to provide the investigator with a clear understanding of the possible risks and adverse reactions, and of the specific tests, observations, and precautions that may be needed for a clinical trial. This understanding should be based on the available physical, chemical, pharmaceutical, pharmacological, toxicological, and clinical information on the investigational product(s). Guidance should also be provided to the clinical investigator on the recognition and treatment of possible overdose and adverse drug reactions that is based on previous human experience and on the pharmacology of the investigational product.

7.4 *Appendix 1:*
TITLE PAGE OF INVESTIGATOR'S BROCHURE (Example)
Sponsor's Name:
Product:
Research Number:
Name(s): Chemical, Generic (if approved)
  Trade Name(s) (if legally permissible and desired by the sponsor)
Edition Number:
Release Date:
Replaces Previous Edition Number:
Date:
7.5 *Appendix 2:*
TABLE OF CONTENTS OF INVESTIGATOR'S BROCHURE (Example)
- Confidentiality Statement (optional)
- Signature Page (optional)
1. Table of Contents
2. Summary
3. Introduction
4. Physical, Chemical, and Pharmaceutical Properties and Formulation
5. Nonclinical Studies
5.1 Nonclinical Pharmacology
5.2 Pharmacokinetics and Product Metabolism in Animals
5.3 Toxicology
6. Effects in Humans
6.1 Pharmacokinetics and Product Metabolism in Humans
6.2 Safety and Efficacy

6.3 Marketing Experience
7. Summary of Data and Guidance for the Investigator
NB: References on
  1. Publications
  2. Reports
  These references should be found at the end of each chapter.
Appendices (if any)
8. *Essential Documents for the Conduct of a Clinical Trial*
8.1 *Introduction*
  Essential Documents are those documents that individually and collectively permit evaluation of the conduct of a trial and the quality of the data produced. These documents serve to demonstrate the compliance of the investigator, sponsor, and monitor with the standards of GCP and with all applicable regulatory requirements.
  Essential Documents also serve a number of other important purposes. Filing essential documents at the investigator/institution and sponsor sites in a timely manner can greatly assist in the successful management of a trial by the investigator, sponsor, and monitor. These documents are also the ones that are usually audited by the sponsor's independent audit function and inspected by the regulatory authority(ies) as part of the process to confirm the validity of the trial conduct and the integrity of data collected.
  The minimum list of essential documents that has been developed follows. The various

documents are grouped in three sections according to the stage of the trial during which they will normally be generated: (1) Before the clinical phase of the trial commences, (2) during the clinical conduct of the trial, and (3) after completion or termination of the trial. A description is given of the purpose of each document, and whether it should be filed in either the investigator/institution or sponsor files, or both. It is acceptable to combine some of the documents, provided the individual elements are readily identifiable.
  Trial master files should be established at the beginning of the trial, both at the investigator/institution's site and at the sponsor's office. A final close-out of a trial can only be done when the monitor has reviewed both investigator/institution and sponsor files and confirmed that all necessary documents are in the appropriate files.
  Any or all of the documents addressed in this guideline may be subject to, and should be available for, audit by the sponsor's auditor and inspection by the regulatory authority(ies).
8.2 *Before the Clinical Phase of the Trial Commences*
  During this planning stage the following documents should be generated and should be on file before the trial formally starts.

	Title of Document	Purpose	Located in Files of	
			Investigator/Institu-tion	Sponsor
8.2.1	Investigator's brochure	To document that relevant and current scientific information about the investigational product has been provided to the investigator	X	X
8.2.2	Signed protocol and amendments, if any, and sample case report form (CRF)	To document investigator and sponsor agreement to the protocol/amendment(s) and CRF	X	X
8.2.3	Information given to trial subject - Informed consent form (Including all applicable translations)	To document the informed consent	X	X
	- Any other written information	To document that subjects will be given appropriate written information (content and wording) to support their ability to give fully informed consent	X	X
	- Advertisement for subject recruitment (if used)	To document that recruitment measures are appropriate and not coercive	X	
8.2.4	Financial aspects of the trial	To document the financial agreement between the investigator/institution and the sponsor for the trial	X	X
8.2.5	Insurance statement (where required)	To document that compensation to subject(s) for trial-related injury will be available	X	X
8.2.6	Signed agreement between involved parties, e.g.:	To document agreements		
	- Investigator/institution and sponsor		X	X
	- Investigator/institution and CRO		X	X (Where required)
	- Sponsor and CRO			X
	- Investigator/institution and authority(ies) (Where required)		X	X

	Title of Document	Purpose	Located in Files of	
			Investigator/Institu-tion	Sponsor
8.2.7	Dated, documented approval/favorable opin-ion of IRB/IEC of the following: - Protocol and any amendments - CRF (if applicable) - Informed consent form(s) - Any other written information to be pro-vided to the subject(s) - Advertisement for subject recruitment (if used) - Subject compensation (if any) - Any other documents given approval/favor-able opinion	To document that the trial has been subject to IRB/IEC review and given approval/fa-vorable opinion. To identify the version number and date of the document(s).	X	X
8.2.8	Institutional review board/independent ethics committee composition	To document that the IRB/IEC is constituted in agreement with GCP	X	X (where required)
8.2.9	Regulatory authority(ies) authorization/ap-proval/notification of protocol (where re-quired)	To document appropriate authorization/ap-proval/notification by the regulatory author-ity(ies) has been obtained prior to initiation of the trial in compliance with the applica-ble regulatory requirement(s)	X (where required)	X (where required)
8.2.10	Curriculum vitae and/or other relevant docu-ments evidencing qualifications of inves-tigator(s) and subinvestigators	To document qualifications and eligibility to conduct trial and/or provide medical super-vision of subjects	X	X
8.2.11	Normal value(s)/range(s) for medical/labora-tory/technical procedure(s) and/or test(s) included in the protocol	To document normal values and/or ranges of the tests	X	X
8.2.12	Medical/laboratory/technical procedures/tests - Certification or - Accreditation or - Established quality control and/or external quality assessment or - Other validation (where required)	To document competence of facility to per-form required test(s), and support reliability of results	X (where required)	X
8.2.13	Sample of label(s) attached to investigational product container(s)	To document compliance with applicable la-beling regulations and appropriateness of instructions provided to the subjects	X	X
8.2.14	Instructions for handling of investigational product(s) and trial-related materials (if not included in protocol or Investigator's Bro-chure)	To document instructions needed to ensure proper storage, packaging, dispensing, and disposition of investigational products and trial-related materials	X	X
8.2.15	Shipping records for investigational prod-uct(s) and trial-related materials	To document shipment dates, batch num-bers, and method of shipment of investiga-tional product(s) and trial-related materials. Allows tracking of product batch, review of shipping conditions, and accountability.	X	X
8.2.16	Certificate(s) of analysis of investigational product(s) shipped	To document identity, purity, and strength of investigational products to be used in the trial.		X
8.2.17	Decoding procedures for blinded trials	To document how, in case of an emergency, identity of blinded investigational product can be revealed without breaking the blind for the remaining subjects' treatment	X	X (third party if ap-plicable)
8.2.18	Master randomization list	To document method for randomization of trial population		X (third party if ap-plicable)
8.2.19	Pretrial monitoring report	To document that the site is suitable for the trial (may be combined with 8.2.20)		X
8.2.20	Trial initiation monitoring report	To document that trial procedures were re-viewed with the investigator and investiga-tor's trial staff (may be combined with 8.2.19)	X	X

8.3 *During the Clinical Conduct of the Trial*
  In addition to having on file the above documents, the following should be added to the files during the trial as evidence that all new relevant information is documented as it becomes available.

246

Appendix D

	Title of Document	Purpose	Located in Files of	
			Investigator/Institution	Sponsor
8.3.1	Investigator's Brochure updates	To document that investigator is informed in a timely manner of relevant information as it becomes available	X	X
8.3.2	Any revisions to: - Protocol/amendment(s) and CRF - Informed consent form - Any other written information provided to subjects - Advertisement for subject recruitment (if used)	To document revisions of these trial-related documents that take effect during trial	X	X

8.3.3	Dated, documented approval/favorable opinion of institutional review board (IRB)/independent ethics committee (IEC) of the following:
	
	- Protocol amendment(s)
	- Revision(s) of:
	  - Informed consent form
	  - Any other written information to be provided to the subject
	  - Advertisement for subject recruitment (if used)
	- Any other documents given approval/favorable opinion
	- Continuing review of trial (see 3.1.4)
		To document that the amendment(s) and/or revision(s) have been subject to IRB/IEC review and were given approval/favorable opinion. To identify the version number and date of the document(s)	X	X

8.3.4	Regulatory authority(ies) authorizations/approvals/notifications where required for: - Protocol amendment(s) and other documents	To document compliance with applicable regulatory requirements	X (where required)	X
8.3.5	Curriculum vitae for new investigator(s) and/or subinvestigators	(See 8.2.10)	X	X
8.3.6	Updates to normal value(s)/range(s) for medical laboratory/technical procedure(s)/test(s) included in the protocol	To document normal values and ranges that are revised during the trial (see 8.2.11)	X	X
8.3.7	Updates of medical/laboratory/technical procedures/tests - Certification or - Accreditation or - Established quality control and/or external quality assessment or - Other validation (where required)	To document that tests remain adequate throughout the trial period (see 8.2.12)	X (where required)	X
8.3.8	Documentation of investigational product(s) and trial-related materials shipment	(See 8.2.15)	X	X
8.3.9	Certificate(s) of analysis for new batches of investigational products	(See 8.2.16)		X
8.3.10	Monitoring visit reports	To document site visits by, and findings of, the monitor		X
8.3.11	Relevant communications other than site visits - Letters - Meeting notes - Notes of telephone calls	To document any agreements or significant discussions regarding trial administration, protocol violations, trial conduct, adverse event (AE) reporting	X	X
8.3.12	Signed informed consent forms	To document that consent is obtained in accordance with GCP and protocol and dated prior to participation of each subject in trial. Also to document direct access permission (see 8.2.3)	X	
8.3.13	Source documents	To document the existence of the subject and substantiate integrity of trial data collected. To include original documents related to the trial, to medical treatment, and history of subject	X	
8.3.14	Signed, dated, and completed case report forms (CRF's)	To document that the investigator or authorized member of the investigator's staff confirms the observations recorded	X (copy)	X (original)

247

	Title of Document	Purpose	Located in Files of	
			Investigator/Institution	Sponsor
8.3.15	Documentation of CRF corrections	To document all changes/additions or corrections made to CRF after initial data were recorded	X (copy)	X (original)
8.3.16	Notification by originating investigator to sponsor of serious adverse events and related reports	Notification by originating investigator to sponsor of serious adverse events and related reports in accordance with 4.11	X	X
8.3.17	Notification by sponsor and/or investigator, where applicable, to regulatory authority(ies) and IRB(s)/IEC(s) of unexpected serious adverse drug reactions and of other safety information	Notification by sponsor and/or investigator, where applicable, to regulatory authorities and IRB(s)/IEC(s) of unexpected serious adverse drug reactions in accordance with 5.17 and 4.11.1 and of other safety information in accordance with 4.11.2 and 5.16.2	X (where required)	X
8.3.18	Notification by sponsor to investigators of safety information	Notification by sponsor to investigators of safety information in accordance with 5.16.2	X	X
8.3.19	Interim or annual reports to IRB/IEC and authority(ies)	Interim or annual reports provided to IRB/IEC in accordance with 4.10 and to authority(ies) in accordance with 5.17.3	X	X (where required)
8.3.20	Subject screening log	To document identification of subjects who entered pretrial screening	X	X (where required)
8.3.21	Subject identification code list	To document that investigator/institution keeps a confidential list of names of all subjects allocated to trial numbers on enrolling in the trial. Allows investigator/institution to reveal identity of any subject	X	
8.3.22	Subject enrollment log	To document chronological enrollment of subjects by trial number	X	
8.3.23	Investigational product(s) accountability at the site	To document that investigational products(s) have been used according to the protocol	X	X
8.3.24	Signature sheet	To document signatures and initials of all persons authorized to make entries and/or corrections on CRF's	X	X
8.3.25	Record of retained body fluids/tissue samples (if any)	To document location and identification of retained samples if assays need to be repeated	X	X

8.4 *After Completion or Termination of the Trial*

After completion or termination of the trial, all of the documents identified in sections 8.2 and 8.3 should be in the file together with the following:

	Title of Document	Purpose	Located in Files of	
			Investigator/Institution	Sponsor
8.4.1	Investigational product(s) accountability at site	To document that the investigational product(s) have been used according to the protocol. To document the final accounting of investigational product(s) received at the site, dispensed to subjects, returned by the subjects, and returned to sponsor	X	X
8.4.2	Documentation of investigational product(s) destruction	To document destruction of unused investigational product(s) by sponsor or at site	X (if destroyed at site)	X
8.4.3	Completed subject identification code list	To permit identification of all subjects enrolled in the trial in case follow-up is required. List should be kept in a confidential manner and for agreed upon time	X	
8.4.4	Audit certificate (if required)	To document that audit was performed (if required) (see 5.19.3(e))		X
8.4.5	Final trial close-out monitoring report	To document that all activities required for trial close-out are completed, and copies of essential documents are held in the appropriate files		X

	Title of Document	Purpose	Located in Files of	
			Investigator/Institution	Sponsor
8.4.6	Treatment allocation and decoding documentation	Returned to sponsor to document any decoding that may have occurred		X
8.4.7	Final report by investigator/institution to IRB/IEC where required, and where applicable, to the regulatory authority(ies) (see 4.13)	To document completion of the trial	X	
8.4.8	Clinical study report (see 5.22)	To document results and interpretation of trial	X (if applicable)	X

Dated: April 30, 1997.

William K. Hubbard,

Associate Commissioner for Policy Coordination.

[FR Doc. 97±12138 Filed 5±8±97; 8:45 am]

BILLING CODE 4160±01±F

Appendix E

FREQUENTLY ASKED QUESTIONS

Frequently Asked Questions About Informed Consent

1. Who may obtain informed consent from patients?

While the principal investigator is ultimately responsible for the informed consent process at his/her site, the investigator may delegate this responsibility to individuals who are knowledgeable about the study and can appropriately present the information and answer questions. (*Code of Federal Regulations (CFR) and International Conference on Harmonization (ICH)*)

2. Who must sign the consent form?

Federal regulations require only that the patient or the patient's legal representative sign and date the consent form before study enrollment. The ICH, some states, and individual Institutional Review Boards (IRBs) require that the person informing the patient and obtaining the consent must also sign the form, and Good Clinical Practice guidelines recommend that the person obtaining consent sign. When a "short form" is used to verify that information from the written summary of the study was presented orally, both the subject and the witness who observed the presentation must sign the short consent form.

3. Can the principal investigator or person obtaining consent sign the consent form after the patient is enrolled?

Since Food and Drug Administration (FDA) regulations do not require the signature of the person obtaining informed consent, it is up to individual IRBs to determine whether this signature is required. However, following Good Clinical Practice guidelines, many consent forms include a place for a dated signature of the person obtaining consent. When it is required (as it is to meet ICH guideline requirements), the person obtaining consent should sign the consent form at the time consent was obtained from the subject.

4. What must be done if changes are made to the consent form reflecting new information or protocol amendments, such as additional information about the investigational treatment, the requirement of additional tests or procedures, or a change in the duration of the study?

- The revised consent form must be approved by the IRB before use.

- The revised and approved consent form must be used to enroll all subsequent patients.

- Previously enrolled patients who have not completed the study treatment period and who will be affected by the changes must be informed and given the opportunity to re-confirm their participation. Documentation that the information or changes were conveyed to patients may be accomplished by having the patient sign revised consent form when applicable. When the new information does not require a consent form, the patient should sign a statement that the information was provided to them.

- For patients who have completed study treatment, information should be conveyed when it refers to safety issues such as potential side effects.

5. What are the IRB's responsibilities for informed consent?

The fundamental purpose of IRB review of informed consent is to assure that the rights and welfare of subjects are protected, and that applicable regulations have been followed. The consent form itself is a written summary of the information that should be provided to subjects, and many investigators use it as a guide for the verbal explanation of the study. The IRB must approve the consent form before the investigator can use it. Because informed consent is a *process*, the consent form serves as an indicator that the investigator is providing patients with appropriate information about the study.

IRBs can implement additional requirements believed necessary to assure informed consent for special communities. These additional requirements may include additional signatures on a consent form, consent form translations, and additional forms for children or other vulnerable subjects.

6. Does the copy of the consent form given to the patient need to be a photocopy of the form with the patient's signature?

This is required by the ICH, some states, and individual IRBs. However, according to the CFR, the copy of the consent form given to the patient can be an unsigned copy of the same consent form signed by the patient.[1] The consent form provides the patient with the opportunity to review the information with others, both before and after the decision to participate, and serves as a continuing reference for the patient, describing study procedures and providing emergency contact names and telephone numbers.

7. Informed consent regulations require the consent form to include a statement that the FDA may inspect the patient records. Is this statement a waiver of the patient's legal right to privacy?

No, the patient does not waive legal rights to privacy. Rather, the FDA requires that patients be informed that complete privacy does not apply in the context of clinical research involving FDA-regulated products. When investigators conduct studies for submission to the FDA, they agree to allow FDA officials access to the study records.[2] Informed consent documents should make it clear that the patient's records automatically become part of the research database, and that patients do not have the option to prevent their records from being reviewed by the FDA. Proper confidentiality procedures are followed when the FDA reviews patient records; however, absolute confidentiality cannot be guaranteed.

8. What is required if a non-English-speaking patient is a potential study subject?

If your site serves an area with a large non-English-speaking population, it would be beneficial to have the consent form translated into the appropriate language before enrollment begins. If a non-English-speaking patient is identified and no written translation is available, an oral presentation must be given in a language understood by the patient. When this occurs, there must be written documentation that the elements of informed consent were orally presented in the appropriate language.

9. What is required if a potential patient is illiterate or physically unable to sign the consent form?

When a patient speaks English but cannot read or write, informed consent can be obtained by having the consent form read verbatim to the patient, and having the patient make a signature mark on the consent form, if allowed under state law. An impartial witness should verify that the process was adequate and that the patient voluntarily consented. If a patient is physically unable to write or make a mark, the patient's legal representative should sign the consent form.

Frequently Asked Questions About Institutional Review Boards (IRBs)

1. **Do IRBs have to be called by that name?**

   No, "IRB" is a generic name used to refer to a group that reviews clinical research and assures the protection of the rights and welfare of the subjects. Each institution may use whatever name it chooses. Regardless of the name chosen, the group is subject to FDA regulations if studies of FDA-regulated products are being reviewed and approved.

2. **Must an institution establish its own IRB?**

   Although not required by the FDA, most institutions participating in clinical research have their own IRBs to oversee research conducted within the institution or by staff of the institution. An institution without an IRB may allow another IRB to be responsible for reviewing and approving studies conducted at the institution. These outside IRBs are often called independent or central IRBs.

3. **What is expedited IRB review?**

   Expedited review allows certain kinds of research to be reviewed and approved without convening a meeting of the IRB members. IRB regulations permit an IRB to review certain categories of research through an expedited process if the research involves minimal risk.[3] The IRB may also use the expedited review process to review minor changes to a previously-approved study during the period covered by the approval. An expedited review may be carried out by the chairperson or by one or more experienced IRB members designated by the chairperson. The reviewer(s) may exercise all the authorities of the IRB except for disapproval, which requires a review by the full committee.

4. **Must an investigator's brochure be included as part of the documents submitted to the IRB for review and approval of a study?**

   For studies conducted under an Investigational New Drug application, an investigator's brochure is usually required.[4] Even though it is not mentioned by name in 21 § CFR Part 56, review of the information contained in such brochures is required.

5. **Are there any regulations that require the investigator to file a report to the IRB when a study is completed?**

   One of the procedural requirements is to ensure the "prompt reporting to the IRB of changes in a research activity."[5] The completion of a study is a change and should be reported to the IRB. Although patients will no longer be at risk since the study is completed, a final report/notice allows the IRB to close its files and provides the IRB with information that may be used in the evaluation and approval of related studies at the institution.

6. **Does an IRB or institution have to compensate patients if injury occurs as a result of participation in clinical research?**

   Institutional policy, not FDA regulation, determines whether compensation and medical treatment will be offered and identifies conditions that might be placed on the compensation and treatments offered. However, the regulations require that if a study involves more than minimal risk, patients *must be told* whether compensation or treatment will be available for research-related injury, and if so, what it is or where further information may be obtained.[6] Statements about the lack of compensation must avoid waiving or appearing to waive any of the patient's rights, or releasing or appearing to release the investigator, sponsor, or institution from liability for negligence.[7]

Frequently Asked Questions About Devices

1. **Why are devices grouped into Class I, Class II, and Class III?**

    The class distinction is based primarily on the level of risk to users/patients and the subsequent level of FDA oversight needed to ensure device safety and effectiveness.

Class I	General Controls	crutches, adhesive bandages
Class II	Special Controls	wheelchairs, tampons
Class III	Pre-Market Approval	heart valves made of new materials

2. **What is the difference between marketing approval under a 510(k) and under a PMA (Pre-Market Approval)?**

    A 510(k) application demonstrates that a new device without a PMA is substantially equivalent to another device that is legally on the market. If the FDA agrees that the new device is substantially equivalent, the device can be marketed.

3. **Why does the IRB have to decide whether a device is Non-Significant Risk (NSR)?**
    The device sponsor/manufacturer makes the initial decision about whether the device carries significant risk to study subjects. If the sponsor believes that the device imparts Significant Risk (SR), the sponsor obtains an Investigational Device Exemption (IDE) from the FDA. Site IRB approval must be obtained before initiating the study.

    If the sponsor/manufacturer believes the device does not impart significant risk, the sponsor does not need to inform the FDA, but does need to have sites obtain IRB approval before the device study can be initiated. If the IRB agrees with the Non-Significant Risk (NSR) assessment, the study may begin and the FDA does not need to be notified. In this sense, the IRB acts as the FDA's surrogate to ensure that the study is conducted safely and in accordance with applicable regulations.

4. **Does the FDA know about an NSR study?**
    As stated in question #3, there is no requirement to report to the FDA when an NSR study starts. However, the requirements for IRB review, informed consent, adverse event reporting, and labeling still apply. Sponsors should be aware, however, that the FDA can later disagree with the NSR determination made by the sponsor/manufacturer and the IRB.

5. **Does the FDA require IRB review of the off-label use of a marketed device?**
    Yes, if the off-label device is to be used in a clinical trial involving human subjects.
    No, if the off-label use is solely used in the practice of medicine, i.e., the physician is treating a patient and no research is being done.

---

[1] 21 CFR 50.27(a) or (b)

[2] 21 CFR 312.68 and 812.145

[3] 21 CFR 56.110

[4] 21 CFR 312.23(a)(5) and 312.55

[5] 21 CFR 56.108(a)(3)

[6] 21 CFR 50.25(a)(6)

[7] 21 CFR 50.20

Appendix F

Form FDA 1572 Instructions for Completing Statement of Investigator Form

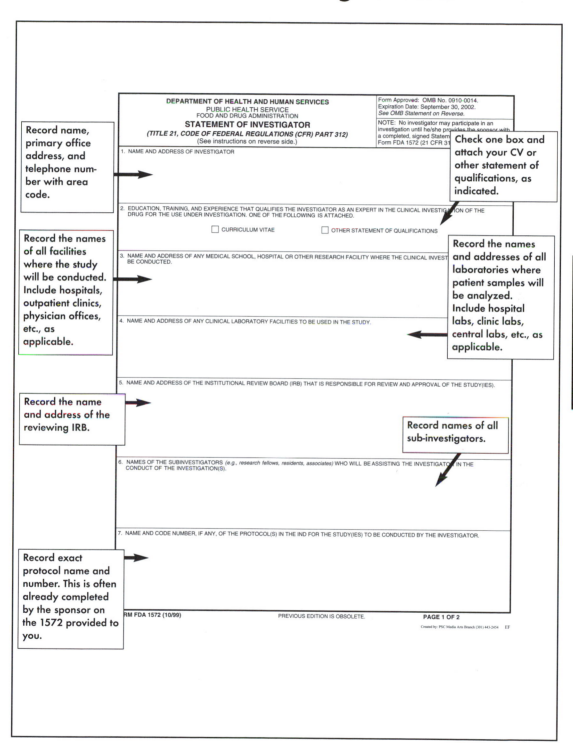

DEPARTMENT OF HEALTH AND HUMAN SERVICES
PUBLIC HEALTH SERVICE
FOOD AND DRUG ADMINISTRATION
STATEMENT OF INVESTIGATOR
(TITLE 21, CODE OF FEDERAL REGULATIONS (CFR) PART 312)
(See instructions on reverse side.)

Form Approved: OMB No. 0910-0014.
Expiration Date: September 30, 2002.
See OMB Statement on Reverse.

NOTE: No investigator may participate in an investigation until he/she provides the sponsor with a completed, signed Statement, Form FDA 1572 (21 CFR 31...

Record name, primary office address, and telephone number with area code.

1. NAME AND ADDRESS OF INVESTIGATOR

Check one box and attach your CV or other statement of qualifications, as indicated.

2. EDUCATION, TRAINING, AND EXPERIENCE THAT QUALIFIES THE INVESTIGATOR AS AN EXPERT IN THE CLINICAL INVESTIGATION OF THE DRUG FOR THE USE UNDER INVESTIGATION. ONE OF THE FOLLOWING IS ATTACHED.

☐ CURRICULUM VITAE   ☐ OTHER STATEMENT OF QUALIFICATIONS

Record the names of all facilities where the study will be conducted. Include hospitals, outpatient clinics, physician offices, etc., as applicable.

3. NAME AND ADDRESS OF ANY MEDICAL SCHOOL, HOSPITAL OR OTHER RESEARCH FACILITY WHERE THE CLINICAL INVEST... BE CONDUCTED.

Record the names and addresses of all laboratories where patient samples will be analyzed. Include hospital labs, clinic labs, central labs, etc., as applicable.

4. NAME AND ADDRESS OF ANY CLINICAL LABORATORY FACILITIES TO BE USED IN THE STUDY.

5. NAME AND ADDRESS OF THE INSTITUTIONAL REVIEW BOARD (IRB) THAT IS RESPONSIBLE FOR REVIEW AND APPROVAL OF THE STUDY(IES).

Record the name and address of the reviewing IRB.

Record names of all sub-investigators.

6. NAMES OF THE SUBINVESTIGATORS (*e.g., research fellows, residents, associates*) WHO WILL BE ASSISTING THE INVESTIGATOR IN THE CONDUCT OF THE INVESTIGATION(S).

7. NAME AND CODE NUMBER, IF ANY, OF THE PROTOCOL(S) IN THE IND FOR THE STUDY(IES) TO BE CONDUCTED BY THE INVESTIGATOR.

Record exact protocol name and number. This is often already completed by the sponsor on the 1572 provided to you.

RM FDA 1572 (10/99)   PREVIOUS EDITION IS OBSOLETE.   PAGE 1 OF 2

Created by: PSC Media Arts Branch (301) 443-2454   EF

Appendix F

Form FDA 1572 Instructions for Completing Statement of Investigator Form

Check applicable box.

ATTACH THE FOLLOWING CLINICAL PROTOCOL INFORMATION:

☐ FOR PHASE 1 INVESTIGATIONS, A GENERAL OUTLINE OF THE PLANNED INVESTIGATION INCLUDING THE ESTIMATED DURATION OF THE STUDY AND THE MAXIMUM NUMBER OF SUBJECTS THAT WILL BE INVOLVED.

☐ FOR PHASE 2 OR 3 INVESTIGATIONS, AN OUTLINE OF THE STUDY PROTOCOL INCLUDING AN APPROXIMATION OF THE NUMBER OF SUBJECTS TO BE TREATED WITH THE DRUG AND THE NUMBER TO BE EMPLOYED AS CONTROLS, IF ANY; THE CLINICAL USES TO BE INVESTIGATED; CHARACTERISTICS OF SUBJECTS BY AGE, SEX, AND CONDITION; THE KIND OF CLINICAL OBSERVATIONS AND LABORATORY TESTS TO BE CONDUCTED; THE ESTIMATED DURATION OF THE STUDY; AND COPIES OR A DESCRIPTION OF CASE REPORT FORMS TO BE USED.

9. COMMITMENTS:

I agree to conduct the study(ies) in accordance with the relevant, current protocol(s) and will only make changes in a protocol after notifying the sponsor, except when necessary to protect the safety, rights, or welfare of subjects.

I agree to personally conduct or supervise the described investigation(s).

I agree to inform any patients, or any persons used as controls, that the drugs are being used for investigational purposes and I will ensure that the requirements relating to obtaining informed consent in 21 CFR Part 50 and institutional review board (IRB) review and approval in 21 CFR Part 56 are met.

I agree to report to the sponsor adverse experiences that occur in the course of the investigation(s) in accordance with 21 CFR 312.64.

I have read and understand the information in the investigator's brochure, including the potential risks and side effects of the drug.

Carefully read this section.

I agree to ensure that all associates, colleagues, and employees assisting in the conduct of the study(ies) are informed about their obligations in meeting the above commitments.

I agree to maintain adequate and accurate records in accordance with 21 CFR 312.62 and to make those records available for inspection in accordance with 21 CFR 312.68.

I will ensure that an IRB that complies with the requirements of 21 CFR Part 56 will be responsible for the initial and continuing review and approval of the clinical investigation. I also agree to promptly report to the IRB all changes in the research activity and all unanticipated problems involving risks to human subjects or others. Additionally, I will not make any changes in the research without IRB approval, except where necessary to eliminate apparent immediate hazards to human subjects.

I agree to comply with all other requirements regarding the obligations of clinical investigators and all other pertinent requirements in 21 CFR Part 312.

INSTRUCTIONS FOR COMPLETING FORM FDA 1572
STATEMENT OF INVESTIGATOR:

1. Complete all sections. Attach a separate page if additional space is needed.

2. Attach curriculum vitae or other statement of qualifications as described in Section 2.

3. Attach protocol outline as described in Section 8.

4. Sign and date below.

An original signature (signature stamps not acceptable) is required. Submit the original Form FDA 1572 and keep a photocopy for your files.

5. FORWARD THE COMPLETED FORM AND ATTACHMENTS TO THE SPONSOR. The sponsor information along with other technical data into an Investigational New Drug Application (IND).

Record date of signature.

10. SIGNATURE OF INVESTIGATOR	11. DATE

(WARNING: A willfully false statement is a criminal offense. U.S.C. Title 18, Sec. 1001.)

Public reporting burden for this collection of information is estimated to average 100 hours per response, including the time for reviewing instructions, searching existing data sources, gathering and maintaining the data needed, and completing reviewing the collection of information. Send comments regarding this burden estimate or any other aspect of this collection of information, including suggestions for reducing this burden to:

Food and Drug Administration
CBER (HFM-99)
1401 Rockville Pike
Rockville, MD 20852-1448

Food and Drug Administration
CDER (HFD-94)
5516 Nicholson Lane
Kensington, MD 20895

"An agency may not conduct or sponsor, and a person is not required to respond to, a collection of information unless it displays a currently valid OMB control number."

Please DO NOT RETURN this application to this address.

FORM FDA 1572 (10/99)   PAGE 2 OF 2

Index

A

Bureau of Chemistry *See* U.S. Bureau of Chemistry

Burroughs-Wellcome Co., 190

C

California, 40

Canada, 37

Cancer, 13, 18

CAP *See* College of American Pathologists

Case Report Forms (CRFs), 72, 75, 84–86, 88–90, 165–166, 182, 185–186, 188

CBER *See* U.S. Center for Biologics Evaluation and Research

CDC *See* U.S. Centers for Disease Control and Prevention

CDER *See* U.S. Center for Drug Evaluation and Research

CDRH *See* U.S. Center for Devices and Radiologic Health

CEC *See* Clinical Endpoints Committee

Center for Biologics Evaluation and Research (CBER) *See* U.S. Center for Biologics Evaluation and Research

Center for Devices and Radiologic Health (CDRH) *See* U.S. Center for Devices and Radiologic Health

Center for Drug Evaluation and Research (CDER) *See* U.S. Center for Drug Evaluation and Research

Centers for Disease Control and Prevention (CDC) *See* U.S. Centers for Disease Control and Prevention

Central institutional review board *See* Institutional review board

CFR *See* U.S. Code of Federal Regulations

Charts, 187

Children *See* Infants and children

Cigarettes, 8

Classes (regulatory), medical device *See* Medical devices

CLIA *See* Clinical Laboratory Improvement Act of 1988

Clinical Endpoints Committee (CEC), 197

Clinical holds, 14

Clinical Laboratory Improvement Act of 1988 (CLIA), 158

CV *See* Curriculum vitae

Cystic fibrosis, 18

D

Dachau (concentration camp), 4

Daniel, Book of (Bible), 2

Data, 90–92, 143–144
  edits, 190–191
  quality, 44, 81, 92
  queries, 44, 86, 165–166, 168, 190–193
  submission, 187–190

Data and safety monitoring, 50

Data and Safety Monitoring Board (DSMB), 120–121, 185

Data and Safety Monitoring Committee (DSMC) *See* Data and Safety Monitoring Board

Data confidentiality *See* Confidentiality

Data edits *See* Data

Data entry/processing, 183

Data forms *See* Patient data forms

Data management, 183–184

Data Monitoring Committee (DMC) *See* Data and Safety Monitoring Board

Data queries *See* Queries

Data worksheets *See* Worksheets

Declaration of Helsinki, 5, 34, 55

Defibrotide, 19

Department of Health and Human Services (HHS) *See* U.S. Department of Health and Human Services

Devices *See* Medical devices

Diaries, 187

Diethylene glycol, 3

Diphtheria, 2

DMC *See* Data and Safety Monitoring Board

DNA, recombinant, 18

Index

F

G

I

Index

K

Kaposi's sarcoma, HIV-associated, 20

Kefauver-Harris Amendment, 5

Kennedy, Pres. John F., 5

L

Labeled (Mis-)
  drinks, 3
  drugs, 3
  foods, 3

Labeling, drug package, 16, 174

Labeling, medical device, 21–22, 25

Laboratories, 34, 126–127, 154, 158, 162

Laboratory certification form, 154, 158

Laboratory normal ranges form, 154, 158

Legislation, Congressional, 2–9

Legislation, local, 34, 36, 39–40, 43, 65

Letter of agreement, 153, 157

Life-threatening diseases, 8

Local factors/laws *See* Legislation, local

M

MAGIC *See* Magnesium in Cardiac Arrest trial

Magnesium in Cardiac Arrest trial, 58

Manufacturers, 34

Massachusetts, 2, 39

Medical Device Amendments of 1976, 6, 22–23

Medical devices, 39, 43–45
  510k, 23–24, 28
  accelerated review, 8

Index

Medical records, 44, 54, 195–196

MedWatch (Medical Products Reporting Program), 29, 41 forms, 30–31

Mentally disabled subjects, 59

Metastatic melanoma, 20

Metastatic renal cell carcinoma, 20

Mexican War, 2

Minority patients, 28, 40

Misbranded
    drinks, 3
    drugs, 3
    foods, 3

Mislabeled
    drinks, 3
    drugs, 3,4
    foods, 3

Monitoring, 79–95, 121

Monitoring logs, 89, 167

Monitoring plans, 50, 84, 87–89, 121

Monitoring visits
    close-out visits, 81, 86–87
    documenting, 89
    initiation visits, 82–84, 87
    on-site, 80–89, 155
    periodic monitoring visits, 81, 84–86
    pre-study visits, 83, 87
    reports, 89

Monitors *See* Study monitors

MPAs *See* Assurances of compliance

Multiple-Project Assurances (MPAs) *See* Assurances of compliance

Index

N

NAI (No Action Indicated), 94

National Commission for the Protection of Human Subjects of Biomedical and Behavioral Research *See* U.S. National Commission for the Protection of Human Subjects of Biomedical and Behavioral Research

National Formulary, 21

National Institutes of Health *See* U.S. National Institutes of Health

National Research Act of 1974, 6

Nazis, 4, 55

NDA *See* New Drug Application

Neonatal respiratory distress syndrome, 20

New Drug Application (NDA), 12, 16, 18, 48, 77, 93, 169, 197

New York, 39

NIH *See* U.S. National Institutes of Health

No Action Indicated (NAI), 94

Non-significant risk devices *See* Medical devices

North Carolina, 190

Notice of Claimed Investigational Exemption for a New Drug *See* Investigational New Drug

Notice of Inspection *See* Form FDA 482

Nuremberg Code, 4, 55

Nuremburg War Crime Trials, 4, 55

Nutritional products, 29–30

O

OAI (Official Action Indicated), 95

Office for Human Research Protections (OHRP) *See* U.S. Office for Human Research Protections

Office for Protection from Research Risks (OPRR) *See* U.S. Office for Protection from Research Risks

Official Action Indicated (OAI), 95

OHRP *See* U.S. Office for Human Research Protections

OPRR *See* U.S. Office for Protection from Research Risks

Organizational chart, 134

Orphan Drug Act of 1983, 7, 20

Orphan drugs, 19–20

P

Package inserts, 16, 68–70

Pasteur, Louis, 13

Patient data forms, 181–197

    Case Report Forms (CRFs), 72, 75, 84–86, 88–90, 165–166, 182, 185–186, 188

    edits, 190–191

    enrollment forms, 185

    follow-up forms, 186, 188

    free text, 184

    paper trail, 182

    patient-completed forms, 187, 193

    queries, 165–166, 168, 190–193

    retention, 169, 197

    safety summary forms, 185, 187

    serious adverse event report forms, 186–187

    worksheets, 182

Patients *See* also Human rights and welfare

    compliance, 145–147

    eligibility, 82–83, 115, 185

    enrollment, 138–140, 142–143, 185

    follow-up, 93, 144–145

    master logs, 164

    patient population, 83, 115, 122–123, 140

    recruitment, 82, 138–140, 154, 163

    screening logs, 164

Penicillin, 3

Periodic monitoring visit checklist, 86–87

Pharmacies, 126

Pharmacopoeia *See* U.S. Pharmacopoeia

Phases *See* Clinical trials

Phocomelia, 5

Pilot trials, 16

PIs *See* Investigators

Pivotal trials, 16, 93

PLA *See* Product License Application

PMA *See* Pre-Market Approval

study design, 113–115, 122

study personnel, 124–126

timelines, 121, 123–124

treatment plan, 115–116

Public Health Service *See* U.S. Public Health Service

Q

QSR *See* Quality System Regulations

Quality assurance audits *See* Site audits

Quality of life, 16, 112–113

Quality System Regulations (QSR), 24

Queries, 86, 165–166, 168, 190–193

Questionnaires, 54, 187, 193

R

Radiologic health, 27

Randomization, 113–114, 142–143

Rare disease/condition devices *See* Medical devices

Rare disease drugs *See* Drugs

Record keeping and retention *See* Clinical trials

Regulations, 34–37

history, 1–9

Regulatory documents, 84, 91

Release of medical information form, 142, 195

Reproduction, human, 13

Research on humans *See* Human rights and welfare

Research subjects *See* Human rights and welfare

Respect (for persons), 6

Roosevelt, Pres. Theodore, 3

S

SAEs (serious adverse events) *See* Adverse events

Safe Medical Devices Act of 1990, 7, 23, 28

Safety and Efficacy Monitoring Committee (SEMC) *See* Data and Safety Monitoring Board

Safety, drug *See* Drugs

Safety letters, 77

Safety, medical device *See* Medical devices

Safety Summary Forms, 185, 187

Sample size, 117

SCD-HeFT *See* Prevention of Sudden Cardiac Death in Heart Failure Trial

Schedule of assessments, 115–116, 122, 129

Screening logs, 164

SEMC *See* Data and Safety Monitoring Board

Serious Adverse Event (SAE) report form 74–76, 85–86, 172, 186–187

Serious adverse events *See* Adverse events

Serums, 6

Shalala, Donna, 98, 101

Signature logs, 166

Signature page *See* Letter of agreement

Significant risk devices *See* Medical devices

Single-project assurances (SPAs) *See* Assurances of compliance

Site audits, 80, 90–91

Site demographics form, 154, 159

Site information sheet *See* Site demographics form

Site inspections, 80, 90–95, 155
    investigator–directed, 90, 93–94
    study–directed, 90, 93

Site Management Organizations (SMOs), 134

Site study team, 135–137

Site visit report, 89

Sites
    adequacy, 81–84
    equipment requirements, 82, 105, 127–128

T

U

U.S. Office for Human Research Protections (OHRP), 9, 51

U.S. Office for Protection from Research Risks (OPRR), 9, 51

U.S. Pharmacopoeia, 21

U.S. Public Health Service, 3, 55

V

Vaccines, 17

development, 2

regulation, 6

VAI (Voluntary Action Indicated), 95

Voluntary Action Indicated (VAI), 95

Volunteers, 15

Vulnerable subjects, 50, 59, 64–65 *See* also Fetuses, Infants and children, Mentally disabled persons, Prisoners, Women

W

Warning Letter, 95

Women, 4, 28, 40

    pregnant, 50, 54, 59, 64

Worksheets, 182, 185

World Medical Association, 5

Index

X

Xenotransplantation, 17–18